The Concise Book of Neuromuscular Therapy

a trigger point manual

The Concise Book of Neuromuscular Therapy

a trigger point manual

John Sharkey

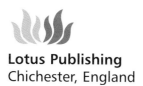

Lotus Publishing
Chichester, England

North Atlantic Books
Berkeley, California

First published in 2008 by
Lotus Publishing
3. Chapel Street, Chichester, PO19 1BU and
North Atlantic Books
P O Box 12327
Berkeley, California 94712

Illustrations Amanda Williams
Text Design Chris Fulcher
Cover Design Jim Wilkie
Printed and Bound in the UK by Scotprint

Acknowledgements

Mention must be made and special thanks given to the wonderful National Training Centre (NTC) tutors of NMT both in Europe and the USA. Thank you to all my students and graduates over the past twenty or so years; it has been a real privilege to teach and learn from you. The author wishes to thank and acknowledge the texts or papers and their authors listed in the resources section, which were invaluable as reference material for the writing of this book.

Dedication

A special thank you to my wife, Fidelma, who has been my greatest supporter and friend without whom this book would never have seen the light of day. Also, to our daughter Xsara who has brought so much love and laughter to our lives. Finally to my friend and colleague Leon Chaitow, thank you.

The Concise Book of Neuromuscular Therapy is sponsored by the Society for the Study of Native Arts and Sciences, a nonprofit educational corporation whose goals are to develop an educational and cross-cultural perspective linking various scientific, social, and artistic fields; to nurture a holistic view of arts, sciences, humanities, and healing; and to publish and distribute literature on the relationship of mind, body, and nature.

British Library Cataloguing in Publication Data
A CIP record for this book is available from the British Library
ISBN 978 1 905367 07 8 (Lotus Publishing)
ISBN 978 1 55643 673 4 (North Atlantic Books)

Library of Congress Cataloging-in-Publication Data

Sharkey, John, MSc.
  The concise book of neuromuscular therapy : a trigger point manual / by
John Sharkey.
     p. ; cm.
  Includes bibliographical references and index.
  Summary: "A manual teaching the techniques of neuromuscular therapy (NMT),
and how to combine it with medical exercise interventions, for the treatment
of soft tissue pain and injury"--Provided by publisher.
  ISBN 978-1-55643-673-4
  1. Manipulation (Therapeutics) 2. Soft tissues injuries--Chiropractic
treatment. 3. Soft tissues injuries--Exercise therapy. I. Title.
  [DNLM: 1. Musculoskeletal Manipulations--methods. 2. Soft Tissue
Injuries--therapy. 3. Holistic Health. 4. Upper Extremity--injuries. WE
805 S531c 2007]
RM724.S33 2007
615.8'2--dc22
                        2007039592

Contents

Foreword   7
About This Book   9
History, Influences, and the Genesis of
Neuromuscular (European) Therapy   11

Chapter 1: Integrated Functional Anatomy:
Building Blocks   15
Understanding Anatomy   17
Prefixes, Suffixes and Combining Forms   18
Anatomical Localization   20
The Cell: Organization of the
Human Body   25
An Overview of the Skeletal System   28
An Overview of the Nervous System   40
An Overview of the
Cardiorespiratory System   43

Chapter 2: Muscles, Fascia, and
the Kinetic Chain   47
Introducing Fascia   48
Planes of Motion   51
Kinetic Chain   53
Classification of Skeletal Muscles and
Muscle Mechanics   53
Titin and the Sliding Filament Theory   70
Muscle Anatomy: Only One Muscle
in the Human Body   71

Chapter 3: Trigger Points:
Assessment and Treatment   79
Trigger Point (TrP) Formation Theories   81
Shoulder Anatomy, Arthrokinematics
and TrP Considerations   85
What is *Proprioception*?   92
Stages of Learning   96

Chapter 4: Kinetic Chain
Anatomy and Patient Assessment   99
Prime Movers, Stabilizers,
and the Kinetic Chain   100
Kinetic Chain Anatomy   101
Looking at Muscle Function   105
Patient Assessment   108
Laws of European
Neuromuscular Therapy   115
Muscle Energy Techniques   118

Chapter 5: Review of the Major
Skeletal Muscles   133
Muscles of the Face, Head, and Neck   134
Muscles of the Trunk   153
Muscles of the Shoulder, Arm, and Hand   167
Muscles of the Hip and Thigh   202
Muscles of the Leg and Foot   218

Resources   229
Index   231

" **I dressed the wound, God healed it .** *"*

Ambroise Paré (1510–1590), was a French surgeon of the Renaissance,
and considered by many as one of the Fathers of Surgery.

Foreword

We are most fortunate to have a pioneer in this field of treatment of musculo-skeletal pain and dysfunctions like John Sharkey to invest so much time and energy in sharing his wealth of experience and expertise with those who are entering the field or want to move a step forward.

I have known John for a number of years and have been deeply impressed by his enthusiasm and effective efforts to promote appreciation and understanding for many neglected aspects of this ubiquitous plague of musculo-skeletal pain and dysfunction in our society and that still is enigmatic to many practitioners. He is dedicated to doing all he can for the multitude of people who suffer unnecessarily because so many health care professionals overlook what is in this book. He has been a good friend who is doing the right things for the right reasons. I cherish him and his enthusiasm. This book marks a high point in John's career at this time.

His focus on neuromuscular therapy recognizes the tight interaction between the muscles and the neuraxis. It keeps in mind the whole person as it looks at individual details. John avoids the current tendency toward microscopic vision where we learn more and more about less and less, becoming so engrossed in the trees that we lose sight of what forest we are in. John has successfully avoided that trap.

Although my career for the past 35 years has been focused on myofascial trigger points and encouraging health care professionals to integrate them into their clinical thinking and practice, I am constantly reminded of the importance of fitting this specialized knowledge into the big picture. The chapter on individual muscles is just right for someone starting out. They supply the information needed clinically without a confusing wealth of detail but still relate to the whole patient.

In the process of deciding what changes to make in my revision of the current myofascial trigger point (MTrP) manuals – that will not become available for about another two years – I decided that each muscle chapter should start with the anatomy first, and then the referred pain patterns. The pain patterns are important but only a part of the diagnostic process. Understanding muscle structure and function is essential for the most effective identification and treatment of muscle pain and dysfunctions.

John has emphasized this important information in this volume. However, what we need to investigate next stems from the fact that the trigger point manuals are only half of the MTrP story. This is of fundamental importance. The current manuals are focused on the pain caused by active MTrPs: the effect of active MTrPs on the sensory nervous system.

What is now becoming apparent is that MTrPs can produce equally potent effects and disturbances in the motor nervous system, causing weakness due to muscle inhibition in the same or other muscles, loss of coordination, and sometimes reflex spasm in other muscles. These distant effects are just about as consistent for a particular MTrP location, and have as much individually variability as referred pain patterns, but are a much different and largely unexplored story. By definition, clinical myofascial pain comes from active MTrPs. Noteworthy, motor disturbances, which usually have no corresponding pain symptoms, are more likely to arise from pain-asymptomatic latent MTrPs that until recently were generally considered just therapeutic red herrings.

You have my heartfelt best wishes for a successful career in this remarkably challenging field.

David G. Simons, MD

About This Book

Neuromuscular therapy (NMT) is a physical (or manual) therapy specializing in the treatment of soft tissue pain and injury (including change in sensation) whilst *medical exercise* aims to provide graded physical activities with specific motor learning sequences to restore functional capacity and reduce the risk of injury occurrence. NMT is innovative in that it combines the best selection of soft tissue manipulation techniques developed by pioneers from a variety of professions such as osteopathy, chiropractic, naturopathy, trigger point therapy, etc. This book aims to provide a description of the underlying principles and concepts of both *neuromuscular therapy* and *medical exercise,* and should be viewed as a teaching aid for the qualified tutor or as a study aid for the student.

This book focuses on the essential anatomy and physiology required to fully understand the underlying science or hypotheses associated with the numerous techniques and physical activities. A description is also provided of the recommended application of the various techniques and a limited number of variations. There is an outline of the rationale concerning the appropriate sequence of neuromuscular therapy and medical exercise interventions with a view to providing a framework within which informed choices can be implemented related to facilitating a patient's return to pain-free movement. In the hands of a qualified therapist, NMT may eliminate the cause of acute or chronic myofascial, muscular, or osseous pain and discomfort. Through the application of the techniques, homeostasis is restored between the nervous, the osseous, and the soft tissue systems.

Neuromuscular therapy enhances the function of joints, muscles, and the general arthrokinematics of the body, and can improve healing by facilitating the return of appropriate core (lumbo-pelvic-hip) muscle function throughout the entire kinetic chain. Special focus is given to the treatment of trigger points, local ischemia, neural interferences, postural and biomechanical dysfunctions, nutritional factors, and emotional wellbeing.

What This Book is not About

This book has not been written to provide the reader with every variation of modality, and will not provide instructions on therapist positioning or hand placements specific to a body part, muscle or group of muscles. I discourage the reader to think that reading this text alone will provide them with the palpatory skills and knowledge needed to ensure appropriate application of neuromuscular therapy. That set of skills and knowledge requires participation in a recognized course of studies under the supervision of a qualified tutor.

Integrated Functional Anatomy: Building Blocks

1

Understanding Anatomy

Prefixes, Suffixes, and Combining Forms

Anatomical Localization

The Cell: Organization of the Human Body

An Overview of the Skeletal System

An Overview of the Nervous System

An Overview of the Cardiorespiratory System

An Integrated Neuromuscular Perspective

The study of anatomy has led to a reductionist view of what is ultimately a *global* or *wholistic* organism. Historically, anatomical study concentrated on specialties, with a focus on specific processes or applications. Anatomists viewed their role as the scientific discipline that investigates the structure of the body including the form of structures, microscopic organization and the process by which they develop. The relationship between structure and function is not always understood. I have written this book to assist the reader to learn the necessary concepts of human anatomy, physiology, exercise science (through medical exercise) and neuromuscular (European) therapy from an integrated perspective.

Regardless of your chosen discipline, whether osteopathy, medical studies, neuromuscular therapy, physiotherapy, physical therapy, chiropractic, massage or other, I want to encourage a change in the way many people think of muscles and movement. A change from single muscle, isolated contractions to many muscles, synergistic, kinetic chain involvement. Not one single note, but a combination of notes resulting in not only a melody, but resulting in a symphony of movement. This is the European neuromuscular perspective.

As you read through the anatomy and neurophysiology presented in this text, I want you to consider the sequence of neuromuscular therapy treatment and phased introduction of medical exercise based on the following model;

1. Injury or insult with resulting protective spasm leads to reciprocal inhibition (altered length-tension curve);

2. Synergistic dominance (altered force couple relationships);

3. Arthrokinetic dysfunction (altered joint motion);

4. Neuromuscular inefficiency;

5. Muscle fatigue (fascial migration);

6. Cumulative injury cycle.

Changes in posture coupled with repetitive movements can be the basis for dysfunction in the myofascial and musculo-skeletal systems and the formation of trigger points. The neuromuscular therapy approach is to achieve optimum neuromuscular efficiency by restoring length-tension relationships, force couple relationships and correct arthrokinetics. When postural alignment is not correct the body will not effectively cope or deal with the forces generated through its tissues.

Rather than being effectively dissipated, these forces will now provide ongoing traumas throughout the myofascial and musculo-skeletal systems not only resulting in faulty movement patterns but causing excessive breakdown and overproduction of tissues. The result is pain and changes in sensations (e.g. numbness, itching, tingling, burning).

This text teaches that certain muscles will shorten when stressed resulting in a switching off of other muscles. This creates muscular imbalances that must first be identified and treated before the patient is encouraged to challenge the muscles through physical activity. Availing of the wonderful techniques of NMT will require an expert understanding of anatomy and so this is where we will start.

Understanding Anatomy

The study of anatomy and physiology is an exciting challenge. In my early student days (I am still a student as study is a lifelong process) the idea of studying anatomy left me in awe. I felt somewhat threatened by the notion that, not only would I have to know about how the body worked, I also needed to learn a new language, the language of anatomy.

It was in the language of anatomy that I found my greatest ally. By investigating the meaning of each new word or term, by breaking down words into their component parts, I removed the threat. I understood in a more profound way.

The word *anatomy* means to dissect, the determination of the regions in an organism that are to be considered its *parts*. Anatomy derives from the Latin *anatomia*, and dissection from the Greek, *anatome*, where *ana* means, *up*, and *temenos* means, *to cut*. This is how anatomists have studied the body for hundreds of years; by cutting. The word *muscle* comes from the word *muscularis* meaning *little mice* (the movement of muscles beneath the skin resembled a mouse moving under a sheet).

The language of anatomy has a wonderful history. Early anatomists, including the father of medicine Hippocrates (460-377BC) and Aristotle (384-322BC) used Latin and Greek terms to describe body parts, prominent structures, muscles, and so on. Hippocrates was a great surgeon whilst Aristotle made accurate observations of adult and embryo animals. Of course Greek and Latin terms are not the only ones used in anatomy. About this time, the medical school in Alexandria, Egypt provided public dissections of human bodies to reveal its internal structures. Many centuries have past since the first recorded descriptions of anatomy in Egypt written on Egyptian papyruses, especially the *Ebers papyrus*, between 3000 and 2500BC (Persand, 1984).

Versalius, including his great piece, *On the Fabric of the Human Body*, revitalized anatomy in the 16th Century. Vesalius and other renaissance anatomists introduced nomenclature, however, and muscles were numbered as a method of study rather than receiving specific names. The method of numbering muscles was introduced by Galen (130–200AD) the greatest physician and anatomist of antiquity and did not change until sometime in the late 17th and early 18th Century when specific myological terminology was used. British anatomist William Cowper and Scottish anatomist James Douglas played no small role in developing named muscles.

Anatomy was progressed by the work of medical students and teachers of universities and medical colleges throughout Europe particularly, Salerno, Padua and Bologna in Italy during the Middle Ages, and at this time the ingenious work of Leonardo da Vinci was born.

The history of anatomy is old and wonderful. If we were to provide names for our muscles today we could say, *the muscle with two tendons on the upper part of the upper limb*. Of course, history has provided us with the term *biceps brachii*, which even sounds poetic. In anatomy, words are often modified with the adding of a prefix or suffix. For example, the suffix 'itis' means inflammation. Tendonitis is therefore the swelling or inflammation of a tendon. By breaking down the words, we can work out the meaning of the anatomical terms or at least have fun trying.

Prefixes, Suffixes and Combining Forms

A good example of a word root, used as a base, is *brachii*, which means *of the arm*. Technically the arm is only from the elbow to the shoulder and below the elbow is the forearm. By adding a prefix at the beginning of a base, or a suffix to the end of a base, you will change its meaning. One can also add a vowel to combine one root to another or to join it with a suffix, known as *combining form*. To assist you to that end here is a list of common prefixes, suffixes, and combining forms with English translation. This will help to remove the threat of learning anatomy. This list is by no means exhaustive, but offers some useful examples. Each example is arranged as follows: alba- (prefix / suffix / combining form); white (translation); e.g. albino (an example where the prefix / suffix / combining form might be used).

a-; without or lacking; e.g. avascular
ab-; away from; e.g. abduct
ad-; to, toward; e.g. adduct
aden-, adeno-; gland; e.g. adenoid
adip-, adipos-; fat; e.g. adipose tissue
aer-, aeros-; air; e.g. aerobic metabolism
af-, ad-; add, move towards; e.g. afferent, adduct
-al-; pertaining to; e.g. brachial
andro-; male; e.g. androgen
angio-; vessel; e.g. angiogram
ante-; in front or before; e.g. anterior
anti-; against or opposed; e.g. antibody
arter-; artery; e.g. arterial
arthro-; joint; e.g. arthrokinetics
-asis; state; e.g. homoeostasis
aur-, auri-; ear; e.g. auricle
auto-; self; e.g. automatic

bi-; two/double; e.g. biceps
bio-; life; e.g. biology
blast-; precursor; e.g. blastocyst
brachi-; arm; e.g. brachialis
bronch-; windpipe/airway; e.g. bronchial
bucc-; cheek; e.g. buccal

calc-; pertaining to the heel; e.g. calcaneus
capit-; head; e.g. capitate
carcin-; cancer; e.g. carcinectomy
cardi-, cardio-; heart; e.g. cardiac
carpal-; wrist; e.g carpal tunnel
cata-; down; e.g. catabolism
caud-; tail; e.g. caudal
cerebr-; brain; e.g. cerebrospinal
chondr-; cartilage; e.g. chondrosis
-cide; destroy, kill; e.g. bactericide
-clast; broken, break, destroys; e.g. osteoclast
con-; together; e.g. connective tissue
contra-; against, opposite; e.g. contralateral
corn-; hard; e.g. cornea
corp-; body; e.g. corpse
cost-; rib; e.g. costal
cranio-; skull; e.g. craniology
crine; to separate; e.g. endocrine

cyst-; sac; e.g. cystoblast
-cyte; hollow cell; e.g. erythrocyte
cyto-; cell; e.g. cytoplasm

de-; away from, down; e.g. detract, depress
dendr-; tree; e.g. dendrite
-derma; skin; e.g. dermabrasion
di-; twice, two; e.g. disaccharide
dia-; through, between, apart, across; e.g. diameter
digit-; finger, toe; e.g. digital
dis-; apart, away from, reversal or separation; e.g. discharge
-duct; draw: e.g. abduct
dys-; painful, difficult, bad; e.g. dysmenorrhea

e-; without, away from; e.g. ebonation
ec-; out from; e.g. eccentric
ecto-; outside (or outer side); e.g. ectoderm
-ectomy; to remove (cut out); e.g. vasectomy
-edema; swelling; e.g. myoedema
-emia; presence of substance in blood; e.g. anaemia
en-; in, into; e.g. endemic
endo-; within, inside; e.g. endomysium
epi-; on, over, above; e.g. epidermis
erythro-; red; e.g. erythrocyte
ex-; out, away from; e.g. exhale
exo-; outside; e.g. exoskeleton
extra-; outside, beyond, in addition; e.g. extracellular

ferent; carry; e.g. efferent
fila-; thread; e.g. filament
form; having shape or form; e.g. fusiform (expressing resemblance)

gastro-, gaster-, gastr-; stomach, belly; e.g. gastrointestinal
-genesis; origin, production, formation; e.g. pathogenesis
glu-; sugar, sweet; e.g. glucose
glyco-; sugar; e.g. glycogen
-gram; a drawing, record of; e.g. myogram
-graph; to write, record; e.g. electrocardiograph

haem-; blood; eg. haematology
hemi-; half; e.g. hemisphere
histo-; tissue; e.g. histology
homeo-; same; e.g. homeostasis
hydro-; water, hydrogen; e.g. hydromassage
hyo-; U-shaped; e.g. hyoid
hyper-; above, more; e.g. hyperactive
hypo-; under, less; e.g. hypoactive

-ia; specified condition; e.g. neuralgia
-iatr-; cure, treat, medical treatment;
e.g. paediatrics
infra-; beneath; e.g. infraorbital
inter-; between; e.g. intervertebral
intra-; within; e.g. intracapsular
ipsi-; itself, same; e.g. ipsilateral
-ism; condition, process; e.g. dimorphism
iso-; equal, alike, uniform; e.g. isometric
-itis; inflammation; e.g. gastritis
kino-, kine-; move, movement; e.g. kinesiology

-lemma; husk, sheath around structure;
e.g. sarcolemma
leuko-; white; e.g. leukocyte
liga-; to bind; e.g. ligament
lipo-; fat; e.g. liposuction

macro-; large; e.g. macrophage
mal-; abnormal, bad; e.g. malalignment
-malaco; soft; e.g. osteomalacia
mega-; big, great; e.g. megacolon
melano-; black; e.g. melanocyte
meso-; middle; e.g. mesoderm
meta-; next, change, after; e.g. metastasis
micro-; small; e.g. microscope
mito-; thread-like, filament; e.g. mitochondria
mono-; one or single; e.g. monosacchride
morph-; form; e.g. morphology
multi-; much, many; e.g. multicellular
myelo; marrow, spinal cord; e.g. myeloid
myo-, muscle; e.g. myocardium

nas-; nose; e.g. nasolacrimal duct
neo-; new; e.g. neonatal
neuro-; nerve, nervous system; e.g. neuromuscular

-oid; form, resemblance; e.g. epidermoid
-ology; the study of science, branch of knowledge;
e.g. physiology
-oma; tumour, swelling; e.g. carcinoma
onco-; mass, tumour; e.g. oncology
orb-; a circle; e.g. orbicularis oris
-ory; referring to; e.g. olfactory
-ose; full of; e.g. adipose

-osis; state, condition; e.g. neurosis, osteoporosis
osteo-; bone; e.g. osteoblast
-ous; expressing material; e.g. serous

para-; near to, beside; e.g. paraplegia
patho-; relationship to disease; e.g. pathology
per-; through; e.g. permeate
peri-; around; e.g. periosteum
phag(o)-; to eat; e.g. phagocyte
-phobia; fear; e.g. hydrophobia
pneumo-; air, lungs, gas; e.g. pneumonia
pod(o); foot; e.g. podiatry
poly-; many, much; e.g. polymer
post-; after, behind; e.g. postpartum
pre-; before, in front of; e.g. prenatal
pseudo-; false; e.g. psendocyst
pterygo-; wing; e.g. pterygoid
pulmo-; lung; e.g. pulmonary

quadr-; four, one quarter; e.g. quadriceps

re-; back, again, contrary; e.g. reabsorption
retro-; backward, located behind;
e.g. retroperitoneal
-rrhagia; burst forth, pour; e.g. menorrhagia
-rrhea; flow, discharge; e.g. amenorrhea

sarco-; flesh; e.g. sarcomere
-sclero-; hard: arteriosclerosis
-sect; to cut; e.g. dissect
semi-; half; e.g. semitendinosus
som-, somato-; body; e.g. somatic
spino-; spine; e.g. spinous process
-stalsis; contractile; e.g. peristalsis
-stasis; stop, stand still; e.g. haemostasis
steno-; a narrowing, contracted; e.g. stenosis
sub-; below; e.g. subcutaneous
super-; above, beyond; e.g. superficial
supra-; above, upon; e.g. supraglenoid
sym-, syn-; together; e.g. symphysis pubis,
synthesis

therm(o)-; heat; e.g. thermoregulation
-thorax; chest; e.g. pneumothorax
-tomy; to cut; e.g. anatomy
trans-; through, across, beyond; e.g. transection
tri-; three; e.g. triceps

-uni; one; e.g. unicellular

vene-; vein; e.g. venesection
vas-; vessel; e.g. vascular
viscer-; internal organ; e.g. viscera

Anatomical Localization

The terms used for anatomical localization are best understood if we think of an animal with a straight central nervous system (i.e. brain and spinal cord), like a lizard. In the case of the lizard the terms rostral, caudal, ventral, and dorsal mean, respectively, towards the rostrum (the nose or face), towards the tail, towards the belly, and towards the back. In humans and other primates, the axis of the central nervous system (CNS) bends, and the face/nose (the rostrum) is no longer at one end of the rostro-caudal axis. Therefore, for the brain, caudal now means towards the back of the head, whilst ventral means towards the body, and dorsal means towards the top of the head.

In the study of anatomy it is normal to study the complex 3-D organization of the CNS through slices. This is called the stereotactic approach (*stereo* from solid object and *tactic* from *tactus*, touch). The most common orientation for slices are axial, a horizontal slice, coronal, a vertical slice that can show both ears, and para-sagittal, a vertical slice that can show from the nose to the back of the head. A sagittal slice is the slice that divides the head in two equal left and right sides. A para-sagittal slice is then any slice parallel to the sagittal slice.

Glossary of Commonly Used Anatomical and Other Terms

All references to human movement are considered to begin from the internationally accepted reference point known as the *anatomical position*. The anatomical position is one of a person standing in an erect position with the face directed forward, the arms hanging by the side, with the fingers extended, and the palms of the hands facing forward: the feet are flat on the ground and slightly turned out. In the anatomical position, joints are said to be in the *neutral position*.

Abduction A movement away from the midline (or to return from adduction).
Acetabulum Meaning 'vinegar bowl'. On the coxal bone, the outer surface presents as a rounded cavity.
Acute Of recent onset (hours, days or a couple of weeks).
Adduction A movement toward the midline (or to return from abduction).
Adhesions Fibroblast formation caused by tearing, or disruption of collagen fibres from trauma, immobilization or as a result of surgical treatment.
Afferent Conveying a fluid or a nerve impulse toward an organ or area (as opposed to efferent).
Analogous Similar in function or appearance but having a different origin or structure (compared with homologous).
Anatomical position The body is upright with the arms and hands turned forward.
Anomaly A structure that is unusual or abnormal.
Anterior Towards the front of the body (as opposed to posterior).
Anterior tilt Anterior tilt rocks the cephalad portion of the pelvis anteriorly with an increase in lumbar lordosis.
Aponeurosis A fibrous sheet of collagenous bundles serving as a connection between a muscle and its attachment.
Articulation A union between two or more bones.

Caudal Directed toward the tail; inferior.
Chronic Long lasting (two weeks or more).
Contralateral On the opposite side.
Coronal plane A vertical plane at right angles to the sagittal plane that divides the body into anterior and posterior portions.
Cranial Relating to/or towards the skull/head.

Deep Away from the surface (as opposed to superficial).
Dermatome An area of skin supplied by a single spinal nerve.

Distal Away from the point of origin of a structure (as opposed to proximal).
Dorsal Relating to the back or posterior portion (as opposed to ventral).

Efferent Conveying a fluid or a nerve impulse away from a central organ (as opposed to afferent).
Evagination To protrude from; an out-pouching, forming a sac or tube.
Extension A movement at a joint resulting in separation of two ventral surfaces (as opposed to flexion).

Fascia Connective tissue lying beneath the skin enveloping muscle groups and investing various organs.
Flexion A movement at a joint resulting in approximation of two ventral surfaces (as opposed to extension).
Foramen A natural opening found primarily in a bone.
Fossa A pit or depression.
Friction A back and forth movement (using digits or other) creating heat in the tissues.
Frontal plane Same as coronal plane.

Ganglion A collection of nerve cell bodies located outside the brain or spinal cord.
Greater trochanter The broad flat process at the top of the lateral femur.

Horizontal plane A transverse plane at right angle to the long axis of the body.

Inferior Below or furthest away from the head.
Insertion The site of an attachment of a muscle, tendon, or aponeurosis to bone.
Intermediate Between two structures.
Ipsilateral On the same side.

Joint The meeting of two or more bones.

Lateral Located away from the midline (opposite to medial).
Ligament A band of fibrous connective tissue joining two or more bones.
Lumen Opening within a tubular organ or vessel.

Meatus A tube like opening within a bone.
Medial Situated close to or at the midline of the body or organ (opposite to lateral).
Median Centrally located, situated in the middle of the body.
Motor Denoting axons that convey impulses from the central nervous system to muscles or glands producing movement or secretion (as opposed to sensory).

Palmar Anterior surface of the hand.
Palpate To examine by pressing or touching.
Para- Prefix denoting along side or next to.
Patent Open or exposed.
Peri- Around or surrounding an object.
Plantar The sole of the foot.
Plexus A network of nerves or vessels.
Posterior Relating to the back or the dorsal aspect of the body (opposite to anterior).
Postganglionic Situated distal to a ganglion.
Preganglionic Situated anterior or proximal to a ganglion.
Prevertebral In front of the vertebral column or vertebrae.
Process A marked prominence protruding from a bone-marking site of attachment of muscles.
Prone Position of the body in which the ventral surface faces down (as opposed to supine).
Proximal Closer to the centre of the body or to the point of attachment of a limb.

Retro- Prefix meaning situated behind.
Rotation Move around a fixed axis.

Sagittal plane A vertical plane extending in an anteroposterior direction dividing the body into right and left parts.

Sensory Axons conveying information from the periphery into the central nervous system (as opposed to motor).

Septum A partition dividing two cavities or masses of soft tissue.

Superficial On or near the surface (as opposed to deep).

Superior Above or closest to the head.

Supine Position of the body in which the ventral surface faces up (as opposed to prone).

Tendon A fibrous band of dense regular connective tissue that attaches a muscle to a bone.

Transverse plane The same as horizontal plane.

Tubercle A small rounded elevation on a bone.

Tuberosity A relatively large protuberance from the surface of a bone.

Valgus position Relates to the alignment of segments of the upper and lower limbs. Position in which the distal bone is abducted with respect to the proximal bone.

Varus position Relates to the alignment of segments of the upper and lower limbs. Position in which the distal bone is adducted with respect to the proximal bone.

Ventral Refers to anterior part of body (as opposed to dorsal).

Regional Areas

The human body is divided into two specific regions known as the *axial* and *appendicular*. The axial division is made up of the head, neck, and trunk. The appendicular division is comprised of the limbs that are attached to the axis of the body. An *axis* is a point around which movement takes place. Figure 1.1a & b shows terms used to indicate specific body areas.

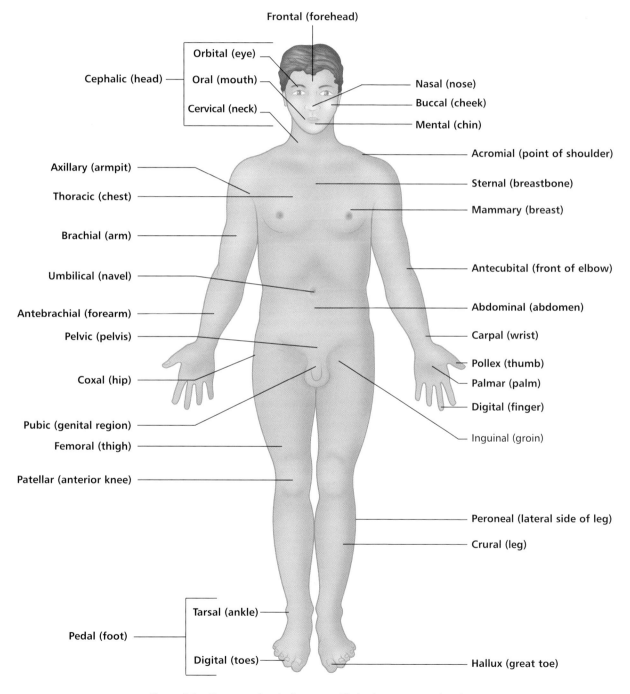

Figure 1.1a: Terms used to indicate specific body areas, anterior view.

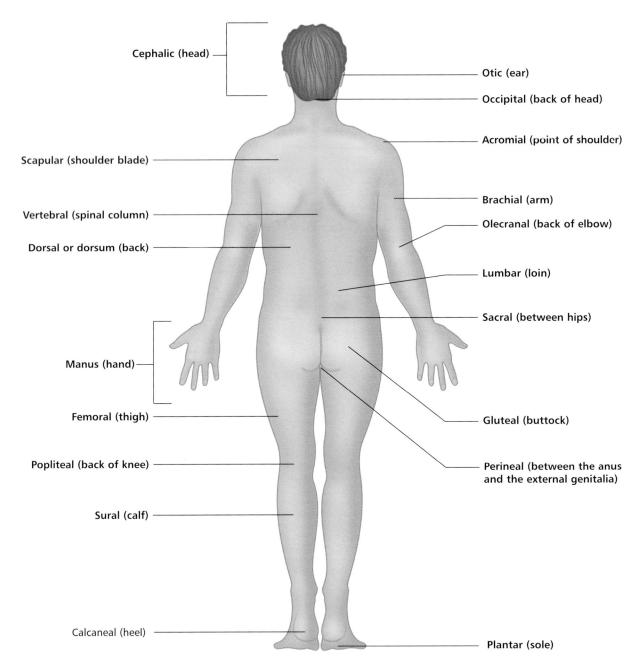

Cephalic (head)

Otic (ear)

Occipital (back of head)

Acromial (point of shoulder)

Scapular (shoulder blade)

Brachial (arm)

Vertebral (spinal column)

Olecranal (back of elbow)

Dorsal or dorsum (back)

Lumbar (loin)

Sacral (between hips)

Manus (hand)

Femoral (thigh)

Gluteal (buttock)

Popliteal (back of knee)

Perineal (between the anus
and the external genitalia)

Sural (calf)

Calcaneal (heel)

Plantar (sole)

Figure 1.1b: Terms used to indicate specific body areas, posterior view.

The Cell: Organization of the Human Body

The simplest form of animal life is made up of a single unit known as a *cell*. Cells got their name as biologists thought that these units resembled small rooms when viewed under a microscope. Specialized cells such as muscle and nerve cells cannot divide and are therefore irreplaceable. Connective tissue cells divide slowly but can also be stimulated to rapid growth when needed. Cells are so crowded with protein organelles, integrins and intercellular matrix, that there is little room for a fluid. Animal cells demonstrate several vital characteristics, which include:

Respiration
All cells need oxygen for combustion with food to provide the energy to carry out its activities. Once energy has been produced by this combustion, carbon dioxide, heat and water will be released into the surrounding fluids of the cell.

Excretion
By-products and waste products will be formed during metabolism. Excretion is the word used to describe the removal of these products from the cell.

Growth
Cells can increase their size by producing additional cellular constituents or making the size of their organelles larger.

Movement
Animal cells can move.

Irritability
Cells can become excited in response to an external stimulus.

Reproduction
Cells, and therefore humans, can replicate themselves, i.e. they can produce new cells. Cells are grouped together to form tissues. Tissues group together to form organs. Organs are grouped together to form an organ system. In anatomy we may speak about the heart, the lungs or the digestive system as separate identities yet none can function without the other. There is of course an inter-linking of all systems, a spillover from one to another.

Eukaryotic Cells
All human cells are *eukaryotic cells*. This means they have a *nucleus*. A covering called the *plasma membrane* surrounds a nucleus. The plasma membrane allows protection so that the internal environment of the cell can act reasonably independently of its surrounding or external environment. The membrane keeps the outside out and the inside in. Cells contain numerous units called *organelles* where the by-products of one enzymatic process are used to provide the energy to fuel another. Cycles occur within these membranes maintaining structural integrity against sudden chemical changes and provide the necessary chemical energy source for cellular activities. Cellular activities require nutrients. The breakdown of these nutrients to provide energy leads to the production of waste products that must be eliminated from the cell.

Our focus will be on activities of the *mitochondria* as they are so important in the production of adenosine triphosphate (ATP). There are more than twenty different types of cells in the human body. Although many anatomy textbooks provide a diagram of a generalized cell (see figure 1.2) there is in fact no such thing. Every cell has a basic structure, which is similar, but their shape and contents are unique to the specific job that each cell must perform.

For example all cells can contract, although muscle cells are better at contracting than other cells. All cells can facilitate nerve signals, but nerve cells do it better than other cells.

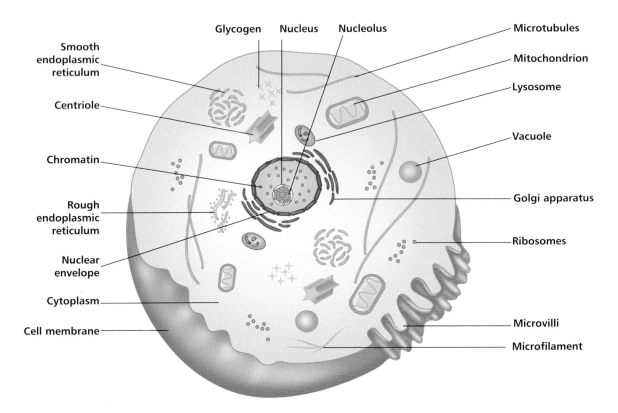

Figure 1.2: A generalized cell.

Cellular Metabolism

All cells require energy to carry out their activities. When you eat anything be it celery, milk, chocolate, meat or bread, these foods must first be broken down into fats, carbohydrates and proteins. These foods are utilized within the body as building materials. After all, you are what you eat. However, if these foods are to be used by our cells to provide energy they must first be broken down at the chemical level to ATP. ATP is the cells exclusive chemical energy source for providing the energy needed to run, think, digest food, to sleep, repair, remodel or whatever.

Cells break down glucose gradually in a series of reactions using small amounts of energy from these reactions to produce ATP. Amongst other things, energy released from these reactions can be used for active transport, synthesis and muscle contractions. ATP is required in large amounts by the cells and as they are constantly using ATP, they must ensure a continuous supply. Of course, making ATP itself requires energy. Let's look at how energy from the breakdown of glucose is used to produce ATP.

Oxidation

Hydrogen transfer is a primary source of energy production as part of a process known as *oxidation*. Using what are called *hydrogen transfer reactions*, pairs of hydrogens are transferred from one substance to another resulting in a release of energy. In cells, hydrogen transfer reactions occur in the mitochondria. Pairs of hydrogens are passed from one substance to another and these substances are called hydrogen carriers. Hydrogen transfer reactions release energy used to make ATP from ADP (adenosine diphosphate). This is made possible by adding a third phosphate to the existing two, thereby creating ATP. These combined processes are known as *oxidative phosphorylation* (OP). OP provides massive quantities of ATP but requires hydrogen from two sources known as *glycolysis* and the *Kreb's cycle*.

Glycolysis

The glucose supplied to the cells from the blood is used to create energy in a process known as *glycolysis*. Glycogenesis and glycogenolysis are the two systems that maintain blood glucose levels. *Glycogenesis* is the production of glycogen from glucose. This is carried out in the skeletal muscles and the liver when blood glucose is too high. *Glycogenolysis* is the opposite of glycolysis. Obviously this occurs when blood glucose levels are low. These two opposite sides of a coin work together to maintain appropriate blood glucose levels at all times.

Oxidative Decarboxylation

The next step in energy production is called *oxidative decarboxylation*. This is strictly an anaerobic process not requiring large amounts of oxygen. Unfortunately when oxygen is in short supply the process of energy production leads to a by-product called *pyruvate*. In this situation pyruvic acids are converted into *lactates*, which are muscle inhibitors. Of course if we did not produce lactic acid we would not know when to slow down or stop. The production of lactic acid could well be seen as a feedback mechanism to protect us from overexertion and even heart attack.

Electron Transport Chain

Finally, provided adequate oxygen is available, fuels go through a series of reactions known as the *electron transport chain* and this continues on to the *Kreb's cycle* (also known as the *citric acid cycle*). In this process fuels are completely broken down with only heat, carbon dioxide and water as the final by products of energy production. Fats, proteins and carbohydrates can all be used as fuels to provide ATP but only when oxygen supplies are sufficient. When oxygen supplies do not meet the current physiological needs of the cells, ATP is produced by anaerobic means. The lack of oxygen dictates that only one fuel source can be used and that fuel is glucose. In this scenario only stored glucose called *glycogen* will be broken down to produce small amounts of ATP. Mitochondria are only involved when there is sufficient supply of oxygen.

It is worth noting that very young children have an immature nervous system that is under development. They do not have the capacity to work effectively anaerobically. This, in effect, means they will not produce sufficient quantities of lactic acid, which is an important negative feedback mechanism to stop the body from overexertion. Some people mistake children, in terms of physiology, as being small adults. This is far from accurate.

Homeostasis

A healthy human must adjust their internal environment constantly, moment to moment, in response to changes in their external environment. Homeostasis (homoio = same, stasis = standing) describes the mechanisms by which a constant internal environment is maintained within certain physiological limits. Homeostasis is disrupted by stresses including injury, trigger points, illness, exercise, emotional state and disease. Control mechanisms are required to ensure homeostasis and this involves feedback systems including proprioceptors. Homeostasis of fluid levels, temperature, gases and blood sugars is essential for positive health and pain free muscles, bones, fascia and joints.

An Overview of the Skeletal System

Functions
The principal functions of the skeleton are mechanical support, movement potential, fat storage, maintenance of calcium homeostasis (including storage), and haematopoiesis in the bone marrow. These functions can be upset in a variety of ways leading to conditions encompassed by the general term, metabolic bone disease. Bone is the hardest tissue in the human body composed of 20% water and 30% organic matter and 50% inorganic matter. Osteoporosis is the commonest metabolic bone disease. Bones are extremely dense connective tissue, in various shapes and sizes offering protection to the soft tissues, including the brain and internal organs.

Bone
Bone cells are contained in cavities known as *lacunae*. Bone cells are surrounded by circular layers of bone matrix that contain collagen and calcium salts. These are needed for healthy bone.

The skeletal system is divided into the *axial skeleton*, including the skull, vertebral column, sternum and ribs, and the *appendicular skeleton*, including the shoulder girdle, the arm and forearm, pelvic girdle and lower limb.

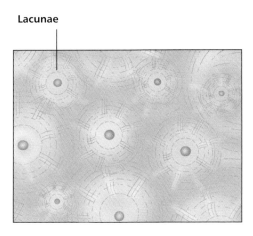

Figure 1.3: Structure of bone.

Cartilage
Cartilage is a type of bone. There are three main types of cartilage in the body, namely;

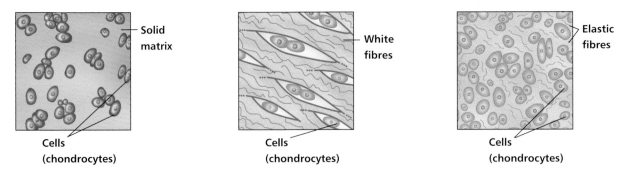

Figure 1.4: Structure of cartilage; a) hyaline cartilage, b) white fibrocartilage, c) yellow elastic cartilage.

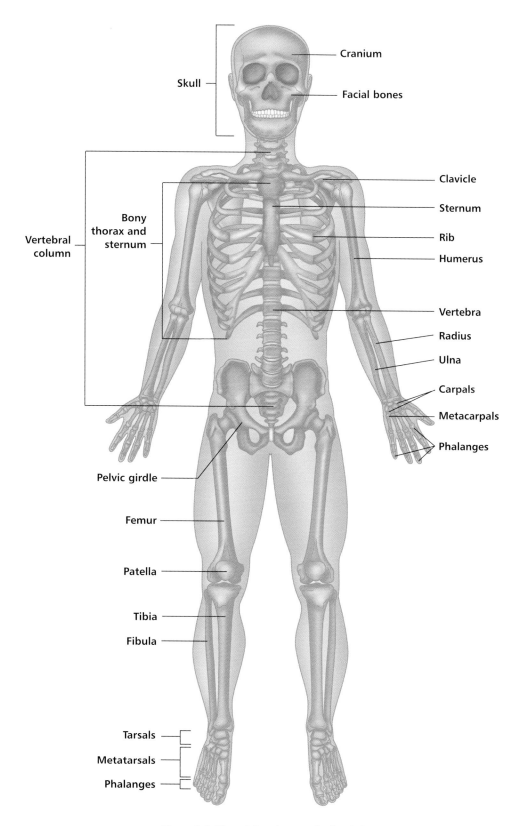

Figure 1.5: The axial and appendicular skeleton.

Classification of Bones

Bones come in many different shapes and sizes, e.g. irregular, flat, short, and long.

Irregular Bones

Irregular bones have complicated shapes; they consist mainly of spongy bone enclosed by thin layers of compact bone. Examples include: some skull bones, the vertebrae, and the hipbones.

Flat Bones

Flat bones are thin, flattened bones, and frequently curved; they have a layer of spongy bone sandwiched between two thin layers of compact bone. Examples include: most of the skull bones, the ribs, and the sternum.

Short Bones

Short bones are generally cube-shaped; consist mostly of spongy (cancellous) bone. Examples include: the carpal bones in the hand, and tarsal bones in the ankle.

Sesamoid bones are a special type of short bone that are formed and embedded within a tendon. Examples are: the patella (kneecap) and the pisiform bone at the medial end of the wrist crease.

Long Bones

Long bones are longer than they are wide; they have a shaft with heads at both ends, and consist mostly of compact bone. Examples include: the bones of the limbs, except those of the wrist, hand, ankle and foot (although the bones of the fingers and toes are effectively miniature long bones).

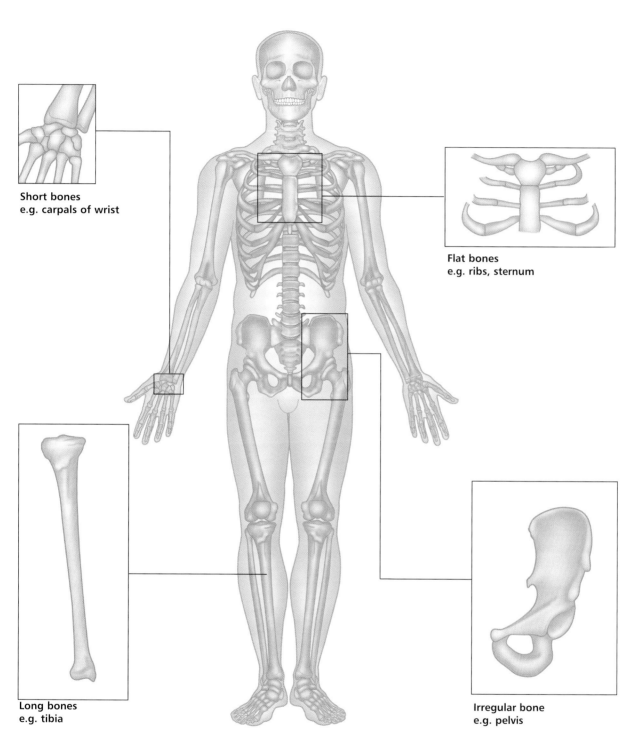

Short bones
e.g. carpals of wrist

Flat bones
e.g. ribs, sternum

Long bones
e.g. tibia

Irregular bone
e.g. pelvis

Figure 1.6: Bone shapes.

Classification of Joints (SAD)

Joints are classified based on the amount of movement available at the joint in conjunction with the anatomy of the joint. Joints do not move at all, move a little, or move a lot.

When we say a joint is *immoveable*, we may mean there is movement but we cannot see this movement with the naked eye. These are classified as **S**ynarthrotic joints. These joints are found mostly in the axial skeleton, where joint stability and firmness are important for the protection of the internal organs. A good example is the joints or sutures in the cranium.

The next classification of joints is referred to as **A**mphiarthrotic. These are *slightly moveable* joints with a layer of fibrous, or cartilaginous tissue between the bones making up the joint. Examples include pubic symphysis, and a sternocostal joint.

Finally, we have **D**iathrotic joints. These joints are also called *freely moveable* or *synovial joints*. Synovial joints have an individual blood and nerve supply, a joint capsule (ligaments) and a synovial membrane with articulating cartilage or meniscus tissue. Examples include: ball-and-socket joint (e.g. shoulder (glenohumeral) joint), and hinge joint (e.g. knee joint).

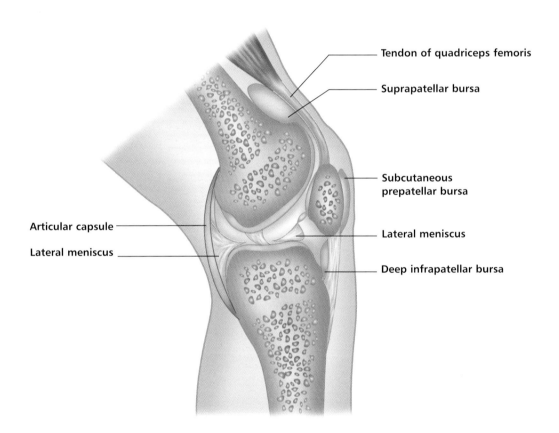

Tendon of quadriceps femoris

Suprapatellar bursa

Subcutaneous prepatellar bursa

Articular capsule

Lateral meniscus

Lateral meniscus

Deep infrapatellar bursa

Figure 1.7a: Shock absorbing and friction-reducing structures of a synovial joint.

The Seven Types of Synovial Joints

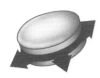

Plane or Gliding
Movement occurs when two, generally flat or slightly curved surfaces glide across one another. Examples: the acromioclavicular joint, and the sacroiliac joint.

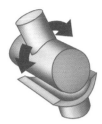

Hinge
Movement occurs around only one axis; a transverse one, as in the hinge of the lid of a box. A protrusion of one bone fits into a concave or cylindrical articular surface of another, permitting flexion and extension. Examples: the interphalangeal joints, the elbow, and the knee.

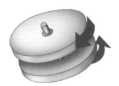

Pivot
Movement takes place around a vertical axis, like the hinge of a gate. A more or less cylindrical articular surface of bone protrudes into and rotates within a ring formed by bone or ligament. Example: the joint between the radius and the ulna at the elbow.

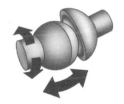

Ball-and-socket
Consists of a 'ball' formed by the spherical or hemispherical head of one bone that rotates within the concave 'socket' of another, allowing flexion, extension, adduction, abduction, circumduction, and rotation. Thus, they are multiaxial and allow the greatest range of movement of all joints. Examples: the shoulder and the hip joints.

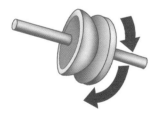

Condyloid
Have a spherical articular surface that fits into a matching concavity. Permits flexion, extension, abduction, adduction, and circumduction. Example: the metacarpophalangeal joints of the fingers (but not the thumb).

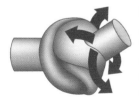

Saddle
Articulating surfaces have convex and concave areas, and so resemble two 'saddles' that join them together by accommodating each other's convex to concave surfaces. Allow even more movement than condyloid joints, for example, allowing the 'opposition' of the thumb to the fingers. Example: the carpometacarpal joint of the thumb.

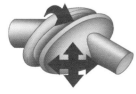

Ellipsoid
An ellipsoid joint is effectively similar to a ball-and-socket joint, but the articular surfaces are ellipsoid instead of spherical, allowing flexion, extension, adduction, abduction, and circumduction. Example: the radiocarpal joint.

Figure 1.7b: The seven types of synovial joints.

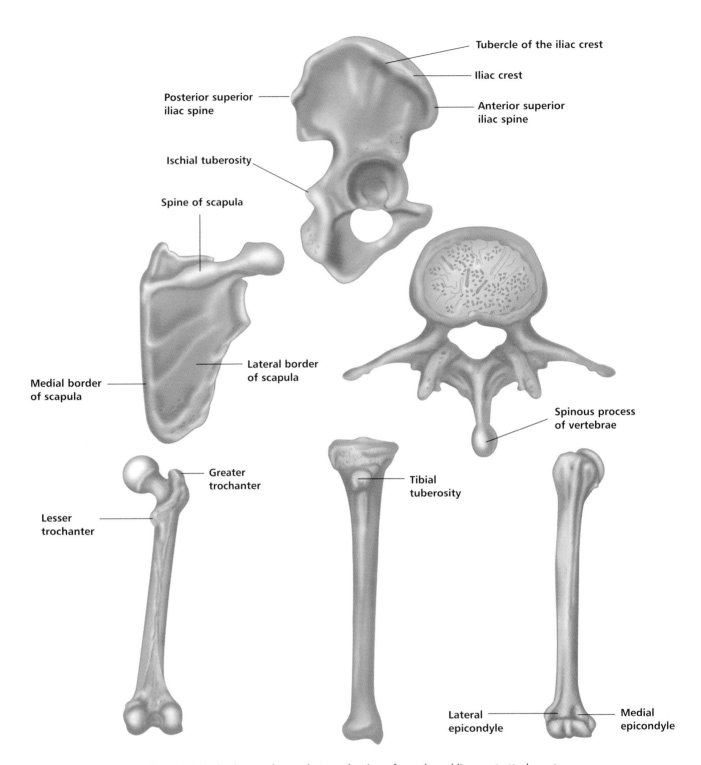

Figure 1.8: Projections on bones that are the sites of muscle and ligament attachment.

Important Bony Landmarks

As muscle is continuous with bone by means of the periosteum, the pulling forces caused by the growth of the bones and the pulling or contractile forces of the muscles and ligaments leads to bumps, lumps, and protrusions. Anatomy has provided special names to describe these. This language helps to establish the origins and insertions of the muscles and ligaments.

Examples include:

Border A narrow ridge of bone.
Condyle A rounded projection forming a joint.
Coracoid A bony projection resembling a crow's beak.
Crest A border or ridge provided by a linear elevation.
Epicondyle A projection over a condyle.
Foramen A hole or opening in bone (or other tissues).
Fossa A shallow depression in a bone.
Mastoid Breastlike or nipplelike.
Notch A narrow gap in a bone.
Process A bony prominence.
Ramus A long branch-like bony continuation of a bone.
Spine A sharp, slight projection.
Styloid A sharp bony projection.
Trochanter A large process on the femur.
Tubercle A rounded blunt and irregular projection.
Tuberosity A large rough and rounded projection.

Although bone is the hardest structure in the human body, it maintains a certain level of elasticity made possible by its structure and composition. Bone is generally enclosed, except in the joint regions where it is coated with articular cartilage, in a fibrous outer dense and vascular fascial membrane called the *periosteum*. Periosteum is composed of two layers, an outer fibrous layer and a deeper elastic layer containing osteoblasts (bone-making cells). These cells are capable of proliferating rapidly when a fracture occurs. In the interior of the long bones is a cylindrical cavity (called the *medullary cavity*) filled with bone marrow and lined with a membrane composed of highly vascular tissue called the *endosteum*. Between these layers is the compact bone or calcium layer. The ends of long bones are known as the *epiphyses* and are filled with red and yellow marrow.

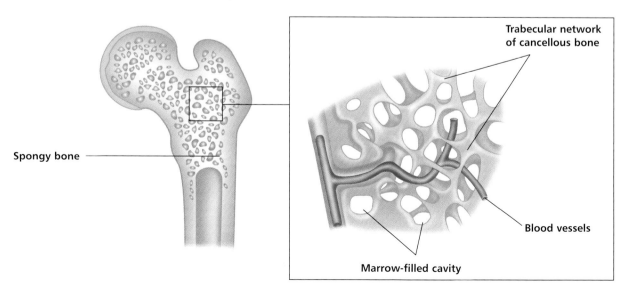

Figure 1.9: Structure of spongy (cancellous) bone.

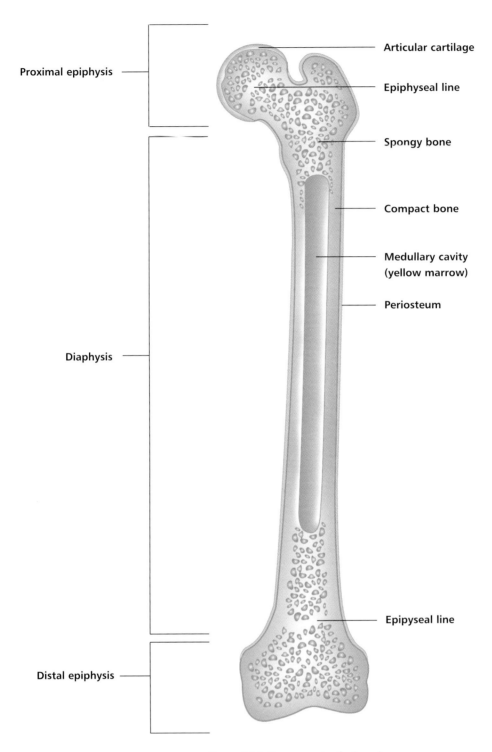

Figure 1.10: Components of a long bone.

Bones are, in general, richly supplied with blood. Blood is supplied by means of *periosteal vessels*. These vessels enter close to the articular surfaces and include nutrient arteries. Canals known as *perforating* or *Volkmann's canals* run at a ninety-degree angle to the long axis of the bone connecting nerve and blood supply within the bone to the periosteum. These canals complete the system of vascular canals in osseous tissue.

Loss of the arterial supply to parts of a bone results in death of bone tissue, usually called *avascular necrosis* or *osteonecrosis*. A number of bones in the body are prone to this complication, usually after injury, including the head of the femur, the scaphoid bone in the wrist, the navicular in the foot and the tibial plateau. Nutrient arteries to the scaphoid bone are large and numerous at the distal end but become sparse and smaller as the proximal end is approached. Fractures of the scaphoid, especially of the waist or proximal end, may be associated with not enough blood being supplied resulting in necrosis and later secondary osteoarthritis. In the foot, the navicular bone is the last tarsal bone to ossify and its ossification centre may be dependent on a single nutrient artery. Compressive forces are thought to be the cause of avascular necrosis of the ossification centre. Trigger points could be another worthwhile consideration as a causative factor.

Athletes tend to have greater bone mineral density, although this effect is often site specific. For example, tennis players have increased bone density in their dominant arm while weight lifters have greater femoral bone density than other athletes. This is consistent with a local effect of exercise on bone. Of course you do not have to be an athlete or a weight lifter. Mild exercise offers many health benefits.

Females who have a total body fat of less than 17% with accompanying amenorrhea are best advised to seek medical advice to ensure the best possible medical care and ensure there is no risk of SHBGs (Serum Hormone Binding Globens). Production of SHBGs can increase the risk of reduced bone health and place even young people at risk of osteoporosis.

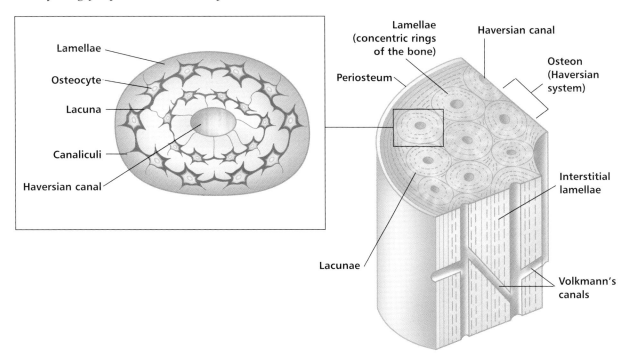

Figure 1.11: Structure of compact bone.

Dietary Influences on Bone Health

Although the majority of body calcium is stored in the skeleton, there has been controversy about the role of dietary calcium intake in the aetiology and prevention of osteoporosis. Published data supports a role for dietary calcium intake in the attainment of peak adult bone density. Poor bone health affects the muscular system and may be a source of trigger point formation. There are a number of dietary factors that play a role in skeletal homeostasis. Sodium intake may have important effects on bone and calcium metabolism. Sodium loading results in increased renal calcium excretion. This has led to the suggestion that lowering dietary sodium intake diminishes age-related bone loss.

Excessive protein and caffeine intake is associated with bone loss. Smoking exposure also has a negative effect on bone health. Poor nutrition includes avoidance of dairy products, and thus a low dietary intake of calcium, or a poor diet overall. Low fat or fat free products are recommended, as are fish, vegetables and water. Professional advice should always be sought from a qualified nutritional expert.

A Little About Connective Tissue

All connective tissue consists of cells and *extracellular matrix* (ECM). The ECM contains insoluble protein fibrils and soluble complexes made up of carbohydrate polymers linked to protein molecules that bind water. From a mechanical viewpoint, the ECM allows the stresses of force and gravity to be distributed ensuring integrity of the shape of the different components of the body. The cells are primarily fibroblastic and produce the ECM.

Connective tissue also contains *macrophages* and *histiocytes*. The ECM of connective tissue consists of three fibre types and ground substance. The fibre types are collagen, elastin and reticulin. The ground substance is a gel-like substance containing the insoluble protein fibrils and soluble complexes made up of carbohydrate polymers linked to protein molecules, which bind water. When the ground substance dries out (due to some stress, overuse insult, injury, etc.) the distance or space between the collagen fibres is compromised allowing adherence to occur resulting in restricted movement. This distance is known as the *critical fibre distance*. Of course dehydration reduces the piezoelectric activity of cells. Whatever facility the cell offers (i.e. contraction, nerve impulse, reproduction, digestion, secretion, etc.) is compromised.

Piezoelectric Activity

The myofascial system at the molecular level is arranged as organic crystalline structures. As such they have the ability to both generate and conduct electrical fields. When a tissue is properly hydrated it will perform its electrical duties more efficiently including ionic bonding, transfer of nutrients and wastes and conducting neural transmissions.

Drawing fluid into the gel-like substance of the ECM, such as when the NMT presses on the tissue, encourages cells to carry out their electrical duties as efficiently as possible. The critical fibre distance is maintained and unrestricted range of motion occurs. Small or micro injuries such as overuse stress initiate the cumulative injury cycle developing inelastic, fibrous adhesions adversely affecting smooth mechanics and tissue extensibility. From the muscular perspective, connective tissue wraps up the muscle tissue and its contractile fibres. There are two primary protein fibres known as *white* and *yellow fibrous tissue*. *Collagen connective tissue (white)*, a strong inelastic compound provides considerable strength without being rigid or elastic. The second, *elastin (yellow)*, is an elastic connective tissue. This highly specialized tissue is capable of considerable deformation yet has the capacity to return to its original shape.

Functions of Connective Tissue

Connective tissue has five main functions:

1. It is a structural frame or scaffolding for all the internal organs and tissues of the human body. It has been described as an *Endless Web*, referring to the spider's web, interwoven throughout the organism providing an elastic rigid structure for the body.

2. Metabolism. Nutrients pass from the capillaries through the connective tissue into cells while by-products of energy production move into the capillaries and lymphatic system.

3. Fighting infections. The removal of dead cells and foreign proteins is facilitated by the connective tissue.

4. Tissue repair. Connective tissue plays a vital role in tissue repair. Fibroblastic activity leads to the deposition of collagenous fibres in damaged tissue to form a scar.

5. Nutrient reservoir. Excessive water, dietary protein, carbohydrates and lipids are all stored in the connective tissue. As fat is stored in the connective tissue this provides vital heat insulation for normal physiological activities.

Types of connective tissue in the skeletal system include osseous tissue, cartilage, periosteum, ligaments, and bone marrow.

An Overview of the Nervous System

The nervous system comprises of two main divisions;

1. The central nervous system consists of the brain and spinal cord.

2. The peripheral nervous system consists of all nerve tissue outside of the spinal cord.

Our nervous system allows us to react and respond to various stimuli.

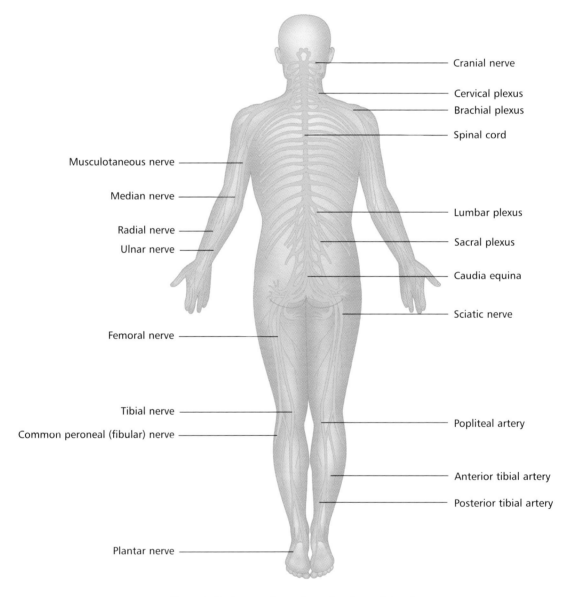

Figure 1.12: A general overview of major peripheral nerves.

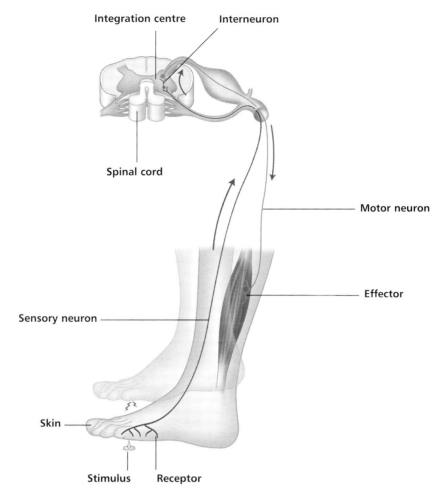

Figure 1.13: Monosynaptic reflex arc.

A stimulus applied to the surface of a cell may result in movement away from or towards the source of the stimulus. Specialized cells called *sensory (afferent)* and *motor (efferent) cells* combine to coordinate our everyday movements. The most relevant sensory organs in NMT include muscle spindles, Golgi tendon organs and receptors that provide detail of pressure, pain, temperature, and position. This information is vital to ensure our muscles can accelerate, decelerate or initiate a reflexive inhibitory response as a protective or facilitating action. For example, your triceps brachii must be inhibited if your biceps brachii is to perform some function requiring flexion at the elbow. If both muscles contracted together no movement would be possible at the elbow joint.

Of course depending on what motion you require, there are times when co-contractions are necessary for a specific movement to occur. In that instance the elbow joint would remain fixed and movement could occur at the shoulder (glenohumeral) joint.

Nervous tissue is composed of *neurons*. Neurons transmit nerve impulses. A neuron is made up an *axon* and a *dendrite*. The axon resembles a long thin wire that arises from the cell body. The dendrites are short protruding fibres that convey impulses towards the cell body.

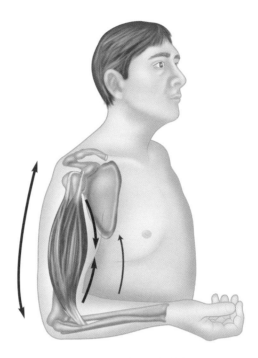

Figure 1.14: Reciprocal inhibition.

The axon can have an outer covering called the *myelin sheath*. The diameter of this fatty covering is constricted at intervals along its length. This tightening or narrowing of the myelin is called the *Nodes of Ranvier*. Axons that have this outer covering are known as myelinated fibres while those without this covering are called unmyelinated. Such fibres are found mostly in the autonomic nervous system. All axons have an outer covering called the *neurolemma* but this is only found on nerves outside the spinal cord.

The nervous system is sending signals to all the body's cells twenty-four hours a day. Neurons that connect the spinal cord (which typically ends between your first and second lumbar vertebrae) to the toes can be as long as half a meter or longer. Nerves can be as thick as your little finger or as thin as a fine thread; in fact they can be microscopic.

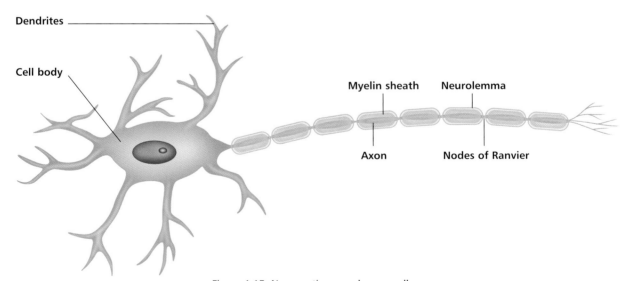

Figure 1.15: Nervous tissue and nerve cells.

An Overview of the Cardiorespiratory System

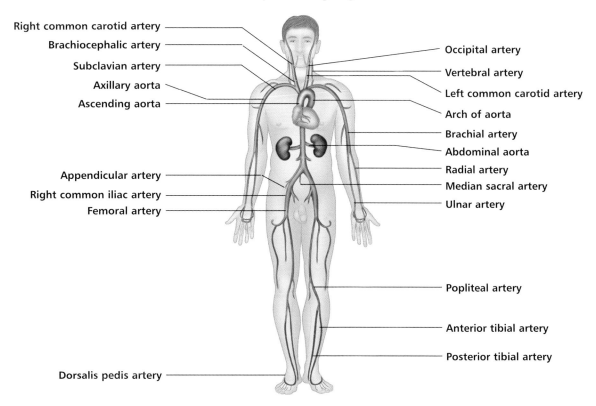

Right common carotid artery
Brachiocephalic artery
Subclavian artery
Axillary aorta
Ascending aorta

Occipital artery
Vertebral artery
Left common carotid artery
Arch of aorta
Brachial artery
Abdominal aorta
Radial artery
Median sacral artery
Ulnar artery

Appendicular artery
Right common iliac artery
Femoral artery

Popliteal artery

Anterior tibial artery

Posterior tibial artery

Dorsalis pedis artery

Figure 1.16: A general overview of major arteries and branches.

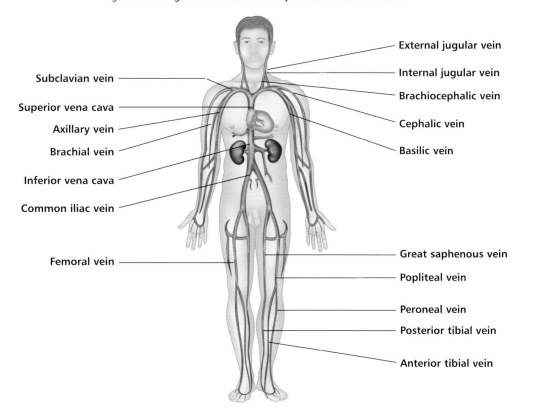

Subclavian vein
Superior vena cava
Axillary vein
Brachial vein
Inferior vena cava
Common iliac vein

External jugular vein
Internal jugular vein
Brachiocephalic vein
Cephalic vein
Basilic vein

Femoral vein

Great saphenous vein
Popliteal vein

Peroneal vein
Posterior tibial vein

Anterior tibial vein

Figure 1.17: A general overview of major veins and branches.

Cardiorespiratory is the term used to describe two systems in one. Of course all the body's systems must work as one. It would be impossible to imagine anyone running on a treadmill for a long time whilst holding his or her breath. They would need to breathe to provide the necessary delivery of oxygen and removal of carbon dioxide. If they did hold their breath they would eventually be forced to take a deep inhalation followed by the need for several more due to oxygen depth. The systems of respiration and circulation need each other. Failure or inefficiency in one will have an effect on the other.

Blood circulates throughout the body in an enclosed one-way system. Blood (a connective tissue) is a thick and bright red liquid that changes colour depending on the quantity of oxygen that it contains. Of course blood always has some oxygen contained in it. It never turns blue, but can look darker, almost rust coloured. Normally the pH of blood is slightly alkaline. Blood volume in the adult male is approximately five litres.

Functions of Blood

1. Transportation. Respiratory gases and nutrients, waste products, hormones, antibodies and more are all moved from one place to another.

2. Protection. White blood cells provide protection against pathogens while platelets provide protection against blood loss through haemorrhage.

3. Regulation. Our body temperature remains close to homeostasis at all times. Blood collects and directs heat throughout the body to where it is needed. When we are producing more heat than required, blood will dissipate the excess by vasodilating blood vessels just beneath the skin.

Components of Blood

Blood is made up of both a solid (living) and liquid (non-living) portion. The solid portion consists of the formed elements erythrocytes (or red blood cells), leukocytes (or white blood cells) and finally thrombocytes (or platelets).

I want to mention the heart and the unique system in place for providing blood to the most important and famous of all blood vessels, the coronary arteries. The heart is a *muscular pump*. It is a muscle containing four chambers that receive and release blood at least once every second at rest. This is known as the *cardiac cycle*. Average heart rates are greater than 70 beats per minute.

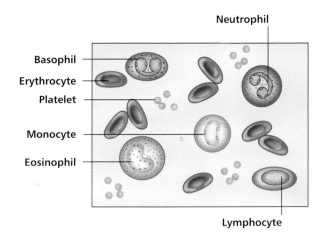

Figure 1.18: Components of blood.

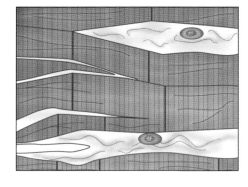

Figure 1.19: Structure of cardiac / striated / involuntary muscle.

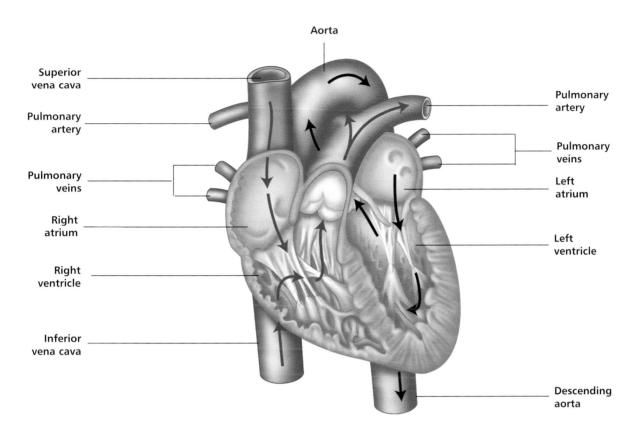

Figure 1.20: The cardiac cycle.

Cardiac Cycle

The cardiac cycle occurs at least once every second. It involves an *active* and *passive* phase. The heart wall or *myocardium* is the muscle part of the heart. It is involuntary and striated. The myocardium requires a supply of nutrient rich blood. The active phase involves the contracting of the myocardium to eject the blood up and out of the chambers. In between beats the heart muscle must relax for a fraction of a second. This is the passive phase when a portion of blood will flow back down the *aorta* into the coronary arteries.

All blood vessels enter and leave the heart from the top. This is an important fact as the aorta, which leaves the left lower chamber (the ventricle), takes ejected blood up towards the head, upper spinal cord and also turns downward to supply the rest of the body (systemic blood supply). What is interesting to know is that this portion of blood will flow backwards in the aorta towards the heart. This back flow occurs during the passive or relaxing portion of the cardiac cycle. The aorta has overlapping valves that ensure this oxygen nutrient blood does not return to the ventricle. These valves allow the blood to pool and collect ensuring a portion will spill into the coronary arteries thus supplying the myocardium.

This vital information supports the need for a gradual warm-up before any physical activity in order to allow the body time to adapt. Sudden shocks to the system increase heart rate and cause vasoconstriction to the coronary arteries. This is turn reduces the passive phase of the cardiac cycle.

Some Useful Terms

Blood pressure The force exerted on the walls of the vessels that contain blood.

Cardiac output The effective volume of blood expelled by either ventricle of the heart per unit of time (usually volume per minute); equal to the stroke volume multiplied by the number of beats (heart rate).

Stroke volume The volume of blood ejected from a ventricle with each beat, equal to the difference between the end-diastolic volume and the end-systolic volume.

Vasoconstriction Reduction in the diameter of blood vessels.

Vasodilation Increase in the diameter of blood vessels.

The combined efforts of the heart, circulatory and respiratory systems maintain the state of *homeostasis* required for an efficient kinetic chain. Homeostasis involves providing the necessary oxygen for cellular activity while ensuring the delivery of appropriate nutrients and removal of by-products. *Ventilation* involves inhaling and exhaling. The chest wall expands and compresses due to muscular and fascial activity including the diaphragm, external intercostals and pleural membranes. The internal intercostal muscles are not involved in quiet normal breathing (this is a passive action based on recoiling of the connective tissues). Only during exertion will accessory muscles take part to increase the thoracic volume and increase the speed at which air is expelled.

Oxygen is necessary for providing the chemical (ATP) needed for energy in sufficient quantity through aerobic pathways. This is the combined function of the circulatory and respiratory system. Failure to provide the internal environment with the correct balance of oxygen and CO_2 results in fatigue, retarded circulation, disturbed sleep, heightened feelings of anxiety and inability to think straight, headaches and painful muscles.

Muscles, Fascia and the Kinetic Chain

2

Introducing Fascia

Planes of Motion

Kinetic Chain

Classification of Skeletal Muscles and Muscle Mechanics

Titin and the Sliding Filament Theory

Muscle Anatomy: Only One Muscle in the Human Body

Introducing Fascia

"Fascia offers a unifying medium, a structure which literally "ties everything together", from the sole of the feet to the meninges which surround the brain. This ubiquitous material offers support, separation and structure to all other soft tissues and because of this produces distant effects whenever dysfunction occurs in it."

Chaitow (1997).

In the late 1970's, Stephen Levin proposed a model for the structure of organic tissue accounting for many physical and clinical characteristics. Levin suggested that all organic tissue must be composed of a type of truss and that the essential building material for all tissues was constructed on the tension icosahedron or the tensegrity model. This is the soft scaffold of the myoskeletal system and forms the basis of the myokinetic chain. The complexities and body wide linkages of the fascia are global. It is an organ of communication.

Dr. Ingber of Boston proposed a model of development control based on tensegrity architecture, in which tissue pattern formation in the embryo is controlled through mechanical interactions between cells and extracellular matrix (ECM) which place the tissue in a state of isometric tension (pre-stress). The model that Dr. Ingber proposed hypothesized that local changes in the mechanical compliance of the ECM, for example, due to regional variations in basement membrane degradation beneath growing epithelium, may result in local stretching of the ECM and associated adherent cells, similar to a 'run in stocking'.

Experiments have established the firm correlation between basement membrane thinning, cell tension generation and new bud and branch formation during tissue morphogenesis and that this process can be inhibited or accelerated by dissipating or enhancing cytoskeletal tension, respectively. This work confirms that mechanical forces generated in the cytoskeleton of individual cells and exerted on the ECM scaffolds, play a critical role in the sculpting of the embryo.

Presently *embryogenesis* (how tissues and organs are formed in the developing embryo) is explained in terms of genes, hormones, and chemical gradients. This is one part of the story. What is important for the professional physical therapist to appreciate, is that while biochemistry and molecular biology have found the power switch that turns on or off different embryological programs by means of specific genes, identification of the light switch on the factory floor does not explain how a finely crafted car is constructed.

It is the micromechanical perspective of the cytoskeleton, how cells sense mechanical forces and convert that information or communication into changes in the intercellular biochemistry and finally into the tissues, the fascia, our posture, joint positioning, and tissue status that is fascinating. Of course these changes are not exclusive to embryogenesis but rather continue throughout our life. The forces we place on our tissues, the fascia, due to repetitive daily tasks or habits (such as sitting, typing, exercising) form and shape the myokinetic fascial system that responds to the tension placed upon it. The end result is your posture, your fascial outline that friends can recognize even at a distance.

Fascia wraps up the viscera, muscles, and even our skeletal system. The fascia of the skeletal system is called the *periosteum* while the fascia covering your visera is the *subserous fascia*. The fascia that lies just beneath the skin (subcutaneous) embraces the entire body from head to toe and is called the *superficial fascia*. The body is a system of interconnecting tubes made of connective tissue fascia including the arterial system, the alimentary system, and the nervous system.

The Largest Organ System

The body possesses an interlocking of fascial planes that connect one muscle group with another. Due to this interconnectedness of the fascial system, restriction in one area will result in reduced range of motion in another local or distal area. The fascia covering the anatomical leg (the *crural fascia*) merges at the inguinal ligament with the *transversalis fascia* wrapping up the *peritoneal cavity*. The *transversalis fascia* merges with the fascia of the diaphragm and continues up to merge with the *parietal pleura* surrounding the lungs. The parietal fascia merges with the *cervical fascia* and on up to the *galea aponeurotica*. This represents the largest organ system in the human body.

The components of the connective tissue mentioned earlier are long, thin, flexible filaments of collagen surrounded by ground substance. The ground substance is made up of glycosaminoglycans (30%) and water (70%), together forming a gel. Acting as a lubricant, this gel maintains the critical fibre distance between the collagen cells. It is easy to visualize that dehydration of the ground substance will adversely affect the free movement of these fibres.

A Little About Fascial Migration

There are typical migration patterns that you will see in most of your patients. Rounded shoulders are a good example. The posterior fascia migrates superiorly and laterally. One can visualize the closing down of the pectoral fascia (anterior) in such a situation. The anterior fascia migrates medially. The elbow and forearm are excellent tools for picking the fascia off the shoulders and gathering up the tissue and slowly moving it medially towards the spine and inferiorly towards the sacrum. Hold the tissue in this position for several breath cycles. The abdominal fascia and lower back can be "hooked" or "scooped" up with the tips of the fingers. When injury occurs or in situations of repetitive stress, fascia becomes tacked down on the periosteum and thickens in the septal spaces between the muscles where it acts as a partition.

The *olecranon* (tip of the elbow) is ideal as a tool to encourage space within these partitions, releasing the three layers of fascia; superficial, middle, and deep. As fascia clings to the periosteum the therapist may feel sand-like particles beneath their fingertips. This tissue should be encouraged away from the bone while asking the patient to gently move the limb or body part involved. Fascial changes can take days, weeks or even years, from the moment of insult, to complete its migration. It is a type of contraction but of course muscles have evolved to be the specialists in that department. Fascial contractions occur at a rate that is not always visible to the eye.

A Little About the Word Dysfunction

When fascia or muscle fibres change their resting status, that is, a muscle fibre shortens or fascia migrates or thickens, we often refer to this as *dysfunction*. In reality, the muscle fibre and fascia are only doing what they are designed to do. Try seeing it as a functional adaptation. The question to ask is, "why is the muscle contracting" or, "why has the fascia migrated".

Fat, Skin and Fascia

Fat is used for several functions including shock absorption, insulation, and energy provision (the capacity to do work) to name but a few. The fatty glycerol contained within the fat cell is, interestingly, encapsulated by fascia. This fascia forms the superficial fascial layer.

I would like to highlight the importance of skin in the role of human movement. The fascia is only one (very important) component of the numerous interactive components of systems within systems within systems. From a simple example it is easy to appreciate that movement at a point where there is a break or tear in the skin would not only be painful but would also further damage the skin as tensile and compressive forces act on the site of the tear causing a larger gap. Research is needed to better appreciate the integrative role that skin plays in providing stability to joints throughout the kinetic chain and assisting in generating and dissipating forces necessary for controlled movements. Apart from the fascia, skin is the largest organ system in the human body and must play a vital role in human movement, a role little understood but with great potential for research.

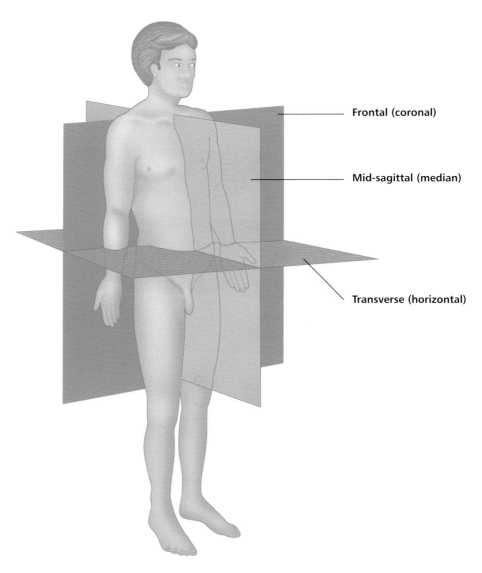

Frontal (coronal)

Mid-sagittal (median)

Transverse (horizontal)

Figure 2.1: Planes of motion.

Planes of Motion

In NMT when we speak of the *kinetic chain*, we are referring to all the body systems as they are linked together in a ubiquitous, continuous system. This text will focus on the relationship of the skeletal, muscular, and nervous systems as they interconnect to generate, absorb, and dissipate forces resulting in human movement.

All human movement takes place on three planes of motion throughout the kinetic chain (see figure 2.1). The kinetic chain must adapt in a synergistic, *body-wide* manner to accept and accommodate the dynamics of functional movement. As the base of support constantly changes the body makes subtle arthrokinematic changes to maintain dynamic balance. Within each plane a single axis can be identified in association with a joint or joints around which movement takes place.

The Mid-sagittal Plane

The *mid-sagittal plane*, also known as the *median plane*, is an imaginary line running vertically through the body moving along an anterior to posterior plane cutting the body into equal right and left sides (also known simply as the *sagittal plane*). Positions *toward* the median plane are called *medial*, and positions *away* from the median plane are called *lateral*. *Ipsilateral* refers to objects on the same side, *contralateral* to objects on the opposite side, and *bilateral* to objects on both sides.

A *sagittal plane* is any plane parallel to the median and hence the median plane is also called the *mid-sagittal plane*. A sagittal slice or section that is not on the median plane is also referred to as a *para-sagittal section*. Any plane running parallel to this line is known as a *para-sagittal plane*.

The Frontal Plane

The *frontal plane*, also known as the *coronal plane*, passes through the body from top to bottom lying at right angles (i.e. perpendicular) to the sagittal plane. This plane divides the body into front (anterior) and back (posterior). The term *posterior* refers to objects on the back half of the body, behind the coronal plane, and the term *anterior* refers to objects in front of this plane.

The Transverse Plane

The *transverse plane*, also known as the *horizontal plane*, is perpendicular to both of these planes and is the plane that divides the body into an upper and a lower half. Positions above the transverse plane are called *superior*, and positions below the transverse plane are called *inferior*. Planes in between these three forming at a 45 degree angle are known as *oblique planes*.

Note: In equine neuromuscular therapy, superior may be called the *rostral* (face or nose) or *cranial* (head) end. Inferior may be referred to as the *caudal* (tail) or *dorsal* (back) ends.

Arthrokinematic Terms

All acts of movement are considered to be a mixture or a single contribution of the following arthrokinematic (arthro – joints, kinematics – movement) terms:

Abduction To move a limb, or body part, away from the midline or to return from adduction. This only applies to movement along the coronal plane.
Adduction To move a limb, or body part, toward the midline. This only applies to movement along the coronal plane.
Circumduction Special combination of movement involving adduction, flexion, extension, and abduction. The resulting movement creates a circular path of movement.
Depression Inferior movement, or moving a body part down, the opposite of elevation.
Elevation Superior movement. To move a body part upwards. This term is often applied to the shoulders (e.g. shrugging the shoulders is elevation).
Extension Opposite of flexion, and there is an increase in the angle. This term applies only to movement along the sagittal or median plane.
Flexion Where there is a reduction in the angle between bones or parts of the body. This term applies only to movement along the sagittal or median plane.
Pronation Rotation of the hand so that the palm faces posteriorly. This is not medial rotation, as this must be performed when the arm is half flexed. Prone means the hand is facing posteriorly.
Protrusion Anterior movement of an object.
Retrusion Opposite of protrusion.
Rotation Movement of an entire limb clockwise (laterally) or anticlockwise (medially).
Supination Rotation of the hand so that the palm faces anteriorly. The hand is supine (facing anteriorly) in the anatomical position.

Special Cases

There are several cases where the meaning of these planes is slightly different. This is apparent in the foot, the tongue, the hand, the brain, and sometimes the perineum.

Foot and Hand

As the foot is discontinuous with the coronal plane, it is described by analogy and with embryological considerations, with the hand.

The palm (*adj.* palmar) of the hand corresponds to the sole (*adj.* plantar) of the foot, and the dorsum (back) of the hand corresponds to the dorsum (top) of the foot.

The term *dorsiflexion* means to flex upwards (true flexion), and the term *plantar flexion* is to extend downwards (true extension).

The term *volar*, used mainly in orthopaedics, is synonymous with *palmar* and *plantar*.

The foot is also capable of movement along another axis due to the flexibility of the ankle joint. These movements are:

1. Eversion. Movement of the sole of the foot away from the median plane.

2. Inversion. Movement of the sole towards the median plane.

The position of the hand in the anatomical position is considered *supine*. Rotation of the hand so that the palm faces backwards is called *pronation*, and the reverse action, *supination*.

Kinetic Chain

European neuromuscular therapy encourages a focus regarding the role of the central nervous system as it shapes and moulds itself through movement experiences to provide the individual with the most efficient selection of muscle synergies. It does this so that a person can perform integrated patterns of movement in the three planes of motion.

The kinetic chain works in a synergistic fashion providing *eccentric* contractions to *decelerate, isometric* contractions to *stabilize* and *concentric* contractions to *accelerate* in three planes of motion. The three planes of movement already mentioned include *sagittal, frontal*, and *transverse* planes and these occur throughout all joints of the kinetic chain. The kinetic chain includes the fascia and all of the body's soft tissues, the periosteum of the skeletal system and finally, the nervous tissues. Therefore, it should include the muscle gastors, tendons, ligaments, the continuous fascia, and the joints involved (arthrokinematics). If one *link* does not operate efficiently due to abuse, overuse, disuse or neural inhibition, the result will involve a change in function and structure throughout the entire *chain*. All tissues contribute to joint stiffness. For example, the joint capsule comprising of the associated ligaments contributes 47%, while the fascia contributes 41%, and tendons provide 10%. Skin provides the remaining 2%.

When a joint is not in correct alignment, tensional force is placed on the associated soft tissues, continuously changing the length tension-relationship of the muscles acting on that joint or joints. This in turn will alter muscle spindle activity, force couple relationships, reciprocal inhibition, and synergistic dominance and decrease neuromuscular efficiency throughout the entire body. To advance knowledge on safe, effective and appropriate physical activities, one must first appreciate the classification of muscles and have an understanding of each of the aforementioned integrated anatomical, physiological, and neurological facilities. The following is a short but informative description of each.

Classification of Skeletal Muscles and Muscle Mechanics

Agonists A muscle that is shortening to perform an action (also known as the *prime mover*) or maintaining a posture.
Antagonists A muscle anatomically opposite to the agonist that can stop or reduce the speed (acceleration) of the agonist (i.e. that is to decelerate).
Neutralizers Muscles, which counteract unwanted actions of secondary or tertiary muscles.
Stabilizers Also known as *fixators*, these muscles contract to offer tension as support to stabilize a body part while a more distal part is moved.
Synergists A muscle that assists the agonist or prime mover to perform a functional movement but is not capable of producing the movement efficiently by itself.

Muscles function together synergistically in force couples to generate force, decrease force, and fixate the kinetic chain. A good example is called *thoraco-lumbar fascia gain*.

In this example, the transversus abdominis (TA), a muscle on the side and front (deep) of the body, contracts to pull the abdominal wall inwards. Acting in a synergistic fashion, the internal oblique (IO) contracts to exert a force on the thoraco-lumbar fascia. This tension has an effect on the second and third lumbar vertebrae causing a lift or extension releasing compression off the fourth and fifth lumbar vertebrae and sacral base. In response to this tension the deep fourth layer muscles including the multifidis and erector spinae contract to offer decelerating forces to trunk flexion and thereby neutralizing the forces of forward flexion. Failure of these muscle synergies, such as in the case of poor core strength, leads to increased lumbar compression, and increased risk of prolapsed or herniated discs. The muscles to target first are those spastic muscles inhibiting the IO and TA. Significant factors (already mentioned) that influence arthrokinematics include: muscle spindles, force couple relationships, reciprocal inhibition, synergistic dominance, neuromuscular efficiency, levers, muscle fibre arrangement (fasciculi arrangement).

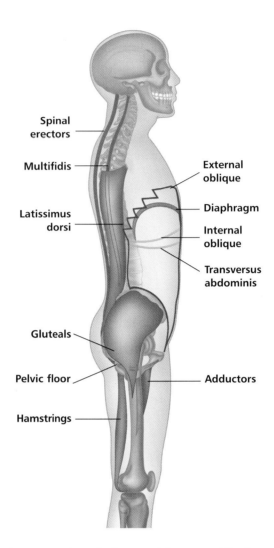

Figure 2.2: Schematic diagram of the core stability (inner unit) muscles, and the global (outer unit) muscles.

Muscle Spindles

Muscles of the human body contain specialized sensory units that are sensitive to muscle lengthening. These sensory units are commonly called *muscle spindles* and their importance in detecting, responding to and modulating changes in the length of muscle is of significant functional importance. An important point to emphasize is that muscle spindles have *three* distinct aspects. Firstly, muscles spindles monitor the *speed* at which a muscle is lengthening. If a muscle is increasing its length with acceleration (speed) the muscle spindles will fire this information to the spinal cord in ratio to the speed at which the muscle is being lengthened. Once this signal reaches the spinal cord, the nervous system is structured in a very specific manner so that the sensory signal travels through an *interneuron* (a connecting cell between a sensory and motor neuron). When the signal has passed through the interneuron it will then pass into a motor neuron and a nerve impulse of equal proportion will travel back to the lengthening muscle, causing it to contract.

As we carry out our daily tasks of walking, climbing stairs, sitting or rising from a chair, our muscles continually receive neural input from spindles that provides the neuromuscular system with a state of readiness or tone.

What is often misunderstood is the second aspect of muscle spindle activity. This is the more static aspect. When a muscle is lengthened and held (i.e. isometrically held, eccentric elongation) it will maintain a contractile response as long as the muscle remains elongated (i.e. stretched). This facility is known as the *stretch reflex* (a monosynaptic reflex arc, see page 41). The static aspect is a *tonic component* while the dynamic, or accelerated aspect, is the *phasic component*.

Muscle spindles will remain irritated or stimulated as long as the stretch is held. The greater the lengths of stretch enforced on a muscle, the more irritated and activated the spindles become.

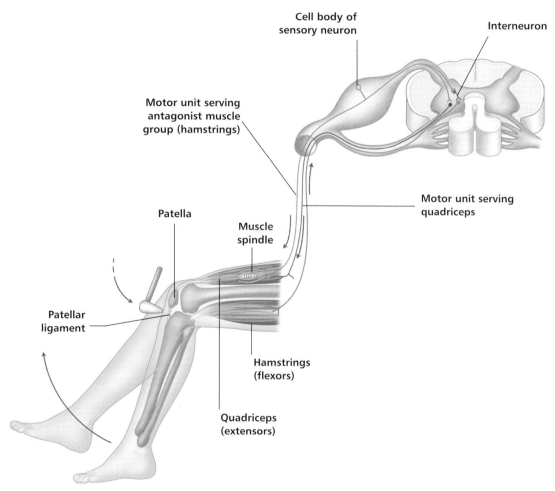

Figure 2.3: The stretch reflex.

The third aspect of muscle spindle activity involves *inhibition*. This involves a neural response resulting in the release of chemicals that inhibit the antagonist muscle to that being stretched. The *patellar tendon stretch* (or *knee jerk test*) is an excellent example of the stretch reflex.

My understanding of these myotactic reflexes has led me to avoid recommending static and ballistic stretching in most situations of physical activity over the past twenty-eight years. As static poses are an integral part of some sports, such as the start of a run or swim, we should not rule out static poses. However, I refer to this as *static dynamic*.

Static stretching may have a therapeutic benefit when used correctly by a knowledgeable and well-trained therapist. Static stretching can cause architectural damage and may interfere with the structural integrity of the connective tissue. Great care is needed to ensure it is the correct intervention to take. The notion that people should be trying to increase range of motion every time they stretch is not one to be supported. The rationale of holding muscles under a static stretch is one that I believe can contribute to increased muscle tension, reduced potential neuromuscular efficiency, and a reduction in relative strength.

In the pursuit of wishing to elongate muscle fibres, I propose that the additional lengthening of nerve tissue could, in turn, result in temporary reduced reaction times while the elongation of muscle fibres disassociates the actin/myosin proteins thereby reducing potential strength and neuromuscular efficiency.

Inappropriate static stretching, I propose, has the potential to pull the walls of individual sarcomeres in opposite directions. This could disassociate the contractile proteins, in many sarcomeres, from each other. In effect this could possibly reduce force output while causing distortion to the sarcomeres in series. Over time, repeated static stretching could lead to increased, or at least maintained, hypertonicity in the muscle. This hypertension becomes self-perpetuating as excessive tension retards both blood and nerve tissues. This retardation leads to tissue hypoxia and additional tissue tension. This in turn may be the foundation for the development of trigger point activity. Many people feel the need to stop and statically stretch their muscles only minutes into their warm-up. Remember warm-up activities should be low in intensity and focused on gradually raising body temperature from the core to the extremities.

Warm-ups should start with small range of motion movements. As blood flow increases to the tissues, fluids begin reducing in viscosity while the muscles and associated fascia become more pliable. Increased temperature augments neural activity and improves diffusion. The exercise selection suitable for warm-ups should not lead to muscle tightness. If it does, a review of the intensity or impact of the exercises is called for. Warm-ups should encourage warm pliable muscles ready for an increase in activity demands, including intensity, range of motion, and duration. Stopping to statically stretch muscles reverses most, if not all, the physiological benefits gained during the warm-up phase. While static stretching is taking place, heart rate and body temperature are dropping while fluid and tissue viscosity is increasing. Respiratory benefits are reversing, nerve augmentation is also reversing…the list continues.

NMT promotes *neuromuscular stretching* or *dynamic range of motion* as well as *spray and stretch* (using ethyl chloride, flouri-methane or similar) as opposed to classical static stretching. It is my recommendation that static stretching has little place in medical exercise, athletic or recreational training.

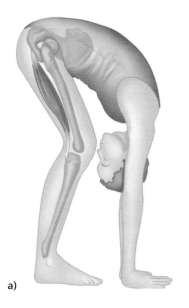
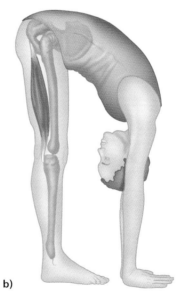

a)   b)

Figure 2.4: a) having to bend the knees to touch the toes is interpreted by many as passive insufficiency of the hamstrings, b) being able to touch the toes with the knees straight would mean there is much less passive insufficiency of the hamstrings.

Static stretching does have a therapeutic role in injury rehabilitation; however, the therapist or trainer must understand how to use static stretching in an appropriate and effective manner. Many fitness experts have promoted static stretching as an effective means of reducing injuries yet time and time again this notion is not supported by research. Many other unsupported claims regarding the benefits of static stretching have also been made. For example, take the *toe touch or sit and reach test*.

These are accepted standard tests for assessing hamstring flexibility. A person deemed to have poor hamstring range of motion or flexibility will bend at the knees as demonstrated in the diagram. Taking into account the posterior kinetic chain tension held in any of the associated 'links' above or below the hamstrings could be the true source of excessive tension. Releasing the plantar fascia in the feet, thoracolumbar or cervical fascia often results in an improved score in any hamstring flexibility test.

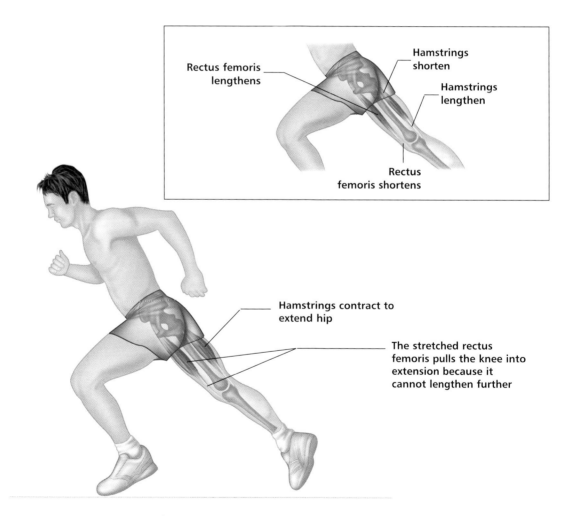

Figure 2.5: Countercurrent movement.

It is my recommendation to all personal trainers, neuromuscular therapists or other physical therapists including physiotherapists, osteopaths, chiropractors, sports therapists, and Rolfers to encourage appropriate warm-ups and cool-downs incorporating gradual increases in range of motion with control. Control involves decelerating towards the end range of movement.

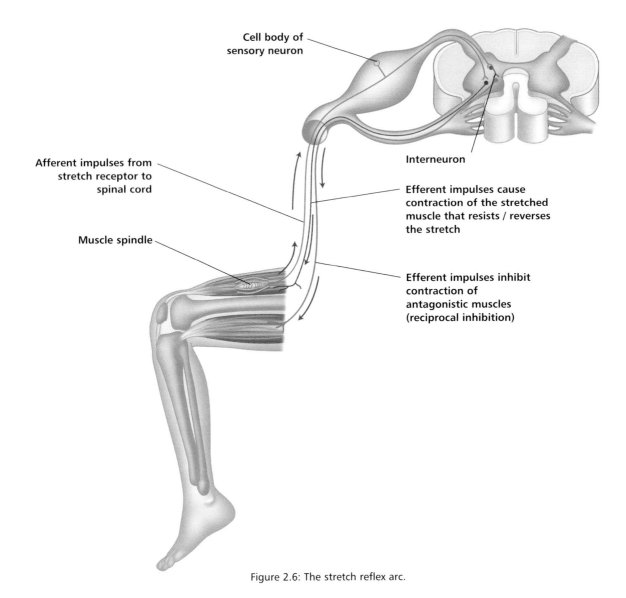

Cell body of
sensory neuron

Interneuron

Afferent impulses from
stretch receptor to
spinal cord

Efferent impulses cause
contraction of the stretched
muscle that resists / reverses
the stretch

Muscle spindle

Efferent impulses inhibit
contraction of
antagonistic muscles
(reciprocal inhibition)

Figure 2.6: The stretch reflex arc.

Recent studies (see references) have shown that static stretching has a negative effect on neuromuscular efficiency including agility and power. Static stretching has been shown to reduce force production in the stretched muscles. In fact, studies have demonstrated that making a fast, dynamic movement following a static stretch increases the risk of injury to that muscle. I want to point out that this is very different to pre-stretching a muscle under load and then immediately following it with a concentric contraction as you would during weight training following an appropriate warm-up. Such a pre-stretch is, by its very nature, dynamic and causes the stretch reflex, thereby, increasing force output.

It is worth noting that recent research regarding proprioceptive neuromuscular facilitation stretching (PNF) has identified increases in electrical activity in the stretched muscles while also increasing muscle stiffness during the stretch. It appears that PNF techniques have a pronounced analgesic effect on the target muscles. This would not be a desired effect for athletes about to engage in high risk, high intensity eccentric actions. Shrier, I. (2004) in his critical review of scientific literature, highlighted that similar to weight training, both force and power decreased immediately after static stretching. The decreases are mild and range from 2–5%. This difference may not be clinically significant for the individual leading a healthy lifestyle but to the elite athlete it may be the difference between first and second place. Of course the debate on stretching must continue and we must be ready to change our views if quality evidence is produced.

Force Couple Relationships

Imagine for a moment you are throwing a ball. As the ball leaves your right hand, your left leg/foot has remained firmly on the ground. Now similar to a DVD, let's freeze that image. A tensional relationship now exists between the opposite lower and upper limbs moving in opposite directions causing a rotation in the vertebral column; this is one example of a *force couple*.

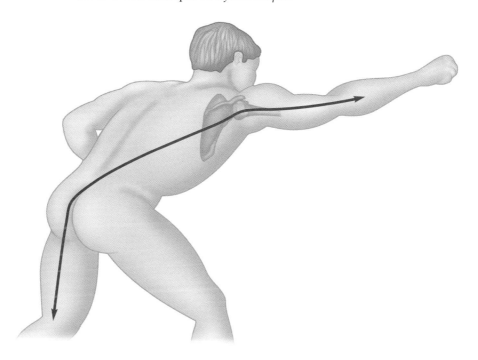

Figure 2.7: Force couple.

Current research supports the benefits of moderate exercise or physical activity in maintaining the health of the musculo-skeletal system. A need exists for a full body kinetic chain postural assessment to be administered before an individualized medical exercise, or physical activity programme can be prescribed. Imagine a client presenting with short *spastic psoas* muscles as one example. Such a scenario would create an inhibition to the *gluteus maximus*. As *gluteus maximus* offers a force couple to the *sacroiliac (SI) joint* in conjunction with *latissimus dorsi* it is easy to see how the *hamstrings* will have to offer additional force, as compensation, to maintain the necessary tension to assist in force closure of the SI joint.

In walking as the left leg is propelled forward, the left ilium rotates backward in relation to the sacrum producing an increase in tension through the sacrotuberous and interosseous ligaments. This helps to provide stiffness, which in turn supports the SI joint, in preparation for heel strike. The ipsilateral hamstrings are activated.

When considering joint biomechanics (arthrokinematics) it is helpful to understand the diversity in degrees of range of motion (ROM) available at various joints. Familiarity with joint ROM will play an important role in the evaluation stage including the kinetic chain postural assessment and the medical exercise prescription. The following are useful examples of normal ROM at the shoulder complex:

Flexion (anteversion)	0 – 180 degrees		Lateral (external) rotation	0 – 80 degrees	
Extension (retroversion)	0 – 50 degrees		Medial (internal) rotation	0 – 100 degrees	
Adduction	0 – 45 degrees		Horizontal extension	0 – 40 degrees	
Abduction	0 – 90 degrees		Horizontal flexion	0 – 140 degrees	
Elevation	90 – 180 degrees				

Key Players

Acceleration Rate of change of velocity with time.

Compression A force that compacts an object.

Displacement The location of one point in relation to another.

Energy The capacity to work, produce motion, overcome resistance, or effect physical change.

Fluid Composed of elements or particles, which freely change their relative positions without separating.

Force A push or pull resulting from physical contact between two objects.

Hydrostatic pressure The intensity of loading within a fluid.

Mass The amount of matter composing an object and the resistance of that object to being moved with speed (i.e. acceleration).

Momentum The mass of an object multiplied by velocity.

Shear Deforms a structure without compacting or stretching it.

Strain Amount of deformity when an object has force applied to it.

Stress Intensity of load equal to the force exerted divided by the area over which it is applied.

Tensile A force which pulls apart.

Velocity Rate of change of displacement with time.

Weight The force acting on an object due to gravitational pull, (e.g. Force + Mass x Acceleration, Newton's Law).

Two Members of the Movement Club

For movement to take place two members, namely *compression* and *tension*, act together to translate generated forces produced by the muscle fibres into orderly, synchronized, adaptable, efficient, and precise movement. The skeletal system, with its joints, provides compression by 'pushing out' while the skin and soft tissues are stretched, activating muscle spindle activity, in turn providing constantly required tension 'pulling in'.

As muscles are integrated into and onto the bones, through the periosteum, their pulling forces generate a tensile stress providing the necessary force to produce tension at a joint. This tension is designed to facilitate movement. In order for movement to occur in a manner that is compatible with the structure of the body, a need exists to avoid creating muscles that *dominate* within a myokinetic chain or link. Training a muscle in a manner that is sagittal plane dominant while focusing on developing strength through large force output is commonplace within the gym setting. This approach to training does little to reduce risk of injury (in fact it may increase risk of injury) as the majority of injuries occur during eccentric movement in the transverse plane.

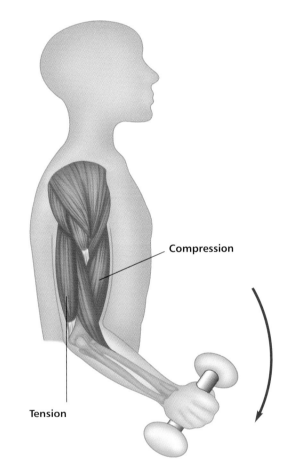

Compression

Tension

Figure 2.8: Two members of the movement club; a) compression, b) tension.

Reciprocal Inhibition

"Few, if any, muscles work in isolation, with most movements involving the combined effort of two or more, with one acting as the prime mover (agonist). Additionally, almost every skeletal muscle has an antagonist (or more than one) that performs the opposite action. Prime movers usually have synergistic muscles which assist them and which contract at almost the same time while their antagonists are quiescent. The agonist(s), synergists and antagonists together comprise the functional unit."

Chaitow, L., & Delany, J. (2002).

Another example of these roles would be hip abduction, in which gluteus medius is the prime mover, with tensor fascia latae acting synergistically and the hip adductors acting as antagonists, being reciprocally inhibited by the action of the agonists.

Reciprocal inhibition (RI) is the physiological phenomenon in which there is an automatic inhibition of a muscle when its antagonist contracts, also known as *Sherrington's Law* (see page 116). Under special circumstances both the agonist and antagonist can contract together, known as a *co-contraction*. An important point to remember is that when a muscle is being inhibited, although the word "relaxed" is used it is not in fact "relaxing". It is receiving a neural impulse to contract but does not do so as it also receives a greater amount of chemical substances that "inhibit" the contraction from occurring. Such substances include phosphates and lactic acid.

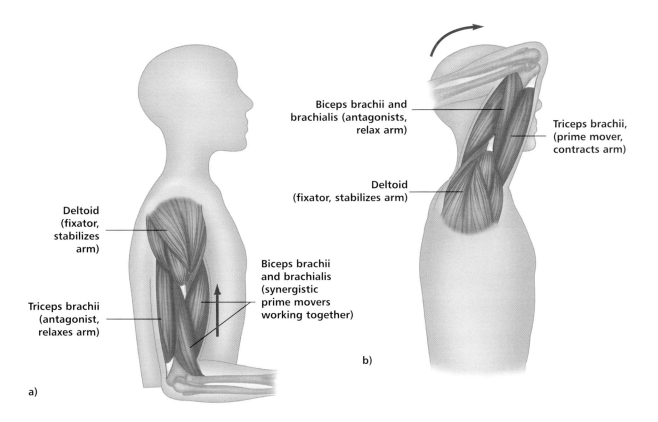

Figure 2.9: Group action of muscles; a) flexing arm at elbow,
b) extending arm at elbow (showing reversed roles of prime mover and antagonist).

Synergistic Dominance

The role of synergists is to assist prime movers to perform functional movements. Due to poor exercise practices, inappropriate posture and repetitive strain on muscles, fascia, and joints, the neural aspects of kinesiology will adapt and change. A kinetic chain reaction both up and down the chain, anterior to posterior, lateral to medial, will occur. If an individual learns to perform an exercise incorrectly, they will always perform that exercise incorrectly. To address this the individual needs to learn correct static and dynamic posture during physical activity. Minute alterations occur in muscle recruitment, stabilization, proprioception and motor skills, strength and joint positioning. Over time this leads to faulty recruitment of muscles within kinetic chains and inhibition of prime movers. When gluteus maximus is inhibited, the synergistic hamstrings and lumbar erectors will inappropriately provide movement of hip extension. Such synergistic dominance could, in time, lead to pain and injury.

Neuromuscular Efficiency

This concerns the capacity of the neuromuscular system to provide safe, effective, and appropriate forces in a synergistic fashion involving agonists, antagonists, synergists, stabilizers, and neutralizers while stabilizing the kinetic chain in all planes of motion. Neuromuscular efficiency takes into account the global effect of movement and the integrated relationship of local muscles (a link) within any given synergy of muscles (a chain), otherwise known as the *integrated functional unit*. Neuromuscular retardation (or reduced efficiency) leads to postural adaptations and increased risk of injury. For example, retardation of reaction time response would increase risk of sprains and strains.

Biomechanics (Arthrokinematics)

Understanding biomechanics is a key element of safe, effective, and appropriate neuromuscular therapy and medical exercise. Aristotle might be considered the first biomechanician, because he wrote the first book on biomechanics called, *De Motu Animalium – On the Movement of Animals*. Along with Socrates and Plato, he identified our most fundamental scientific tools: deductive reasoning, and mathematical reasoning and so biomechanics was born.

Muscle Fibre Arrangement (Fasciculi Arrangement)

Muscles pull, they cannot push. Of course that means that you use the same muscles to pick up your shopping bags as you do to put them down again. If you can imagine a person sitting in a pec deck exercise machine, although the person pushes the pads away from their body, it is in fact the pulling action of the pectoralis and associated muscles that provide the "pulling" force to overcome the resistance. Muscles can only provide forces in the direction that their muscle fibres are running. In NMT this is known as *directional force* or *line of pull*. Muscles have three classifications:

1. Skeletal muscle, also known as striated or voluntary muscle, is under direct nervous control. Skeletal muscles fatigue easily, but can be strengthened. They are capable of powerful, rapid contractions, and longer, sustained contractions. This contractile body (the muscle proper) is usually attached to two bony points. Attachments may be either, tendinous, by aponeurosis, or by raphe.

2. Cardiac muscle is also striated, but is confined to the heart, and is under involuntary nervous control.

3. Smooth muscle, also known as visceral muscle, is like cardiac muscle, and under involuntary nervous control. It is found in the walls of the alimentary tract, blood vessels, and stomach, and provides a slow and sustained response (i.e. contraction). Smooth muscle is usually seen as flat sheets, sometimes wrapped around an internal organ like a gut in circular and longitudinal layers, or arranged as a sphincter to close off a tube (as in the opening to the stomach).

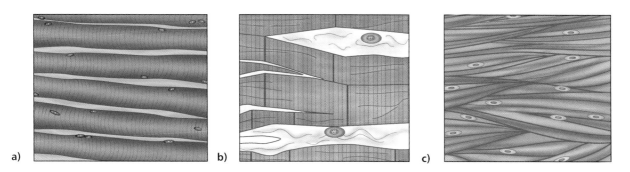

Figure 2.10: Structure of muscle; a) skeletal muscle, b) cardiac muscle, c) smooth muscle.

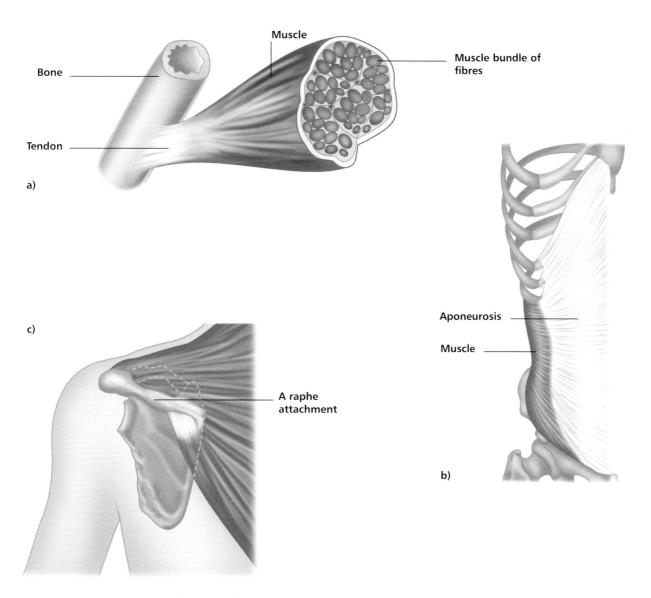

Figure 2.11: Attachments by, a) tendon, b) aponeurosis, c) raphe.

Tendons are an integral part and continuation of muscle. The tendon is a fibrous band of tissue that is flexible enough to bend around bones and joints. It is avascular and therefore appears white in colour and heals very slowly. Tendons take the form of cords or strips, circular in cross section, oval or flattened. They are made up of bundles (*fascicles*) of collagen fibres, mostly parallel. Surrounding the outside is an *epitendineum* with elastic fibres, which causes a little drag as tendons run through connective tissue. Where they have to move independently of other tissues, various friction-reducing devices are used. The tendon may run over *cartilage*, or over a *sesamoid bone*, such as the patella, or a *bursa* may be interposed. This bursa may be elongated and folded around the tendon to form a sheath. As mentioned, a flattened tendon is an *aponeurosis*.

A *raphe* attachment is a fleshy insertion joining muscle to bone without the intervention of a collagenous tendon or aponeurosis. The collagen is still there among the muscle fibres, or forming a very short tendon.

Origins and Insertions
Muscles are often said to have an *origin* at one end and an *insertion* at the other. The origin (the one that moves least on contraction) is often proximal, with the insertion distal. Origins and insertions can change their role depending on the body's position relative to gravity. As this is the case we can also refer to muscle attachments as opposed to origins and insertions if preferred. Many times a muscle originates from more than one place: it is then said to have two heads (e.g. biceps brachii) or three heads (e.g. triceps brachii).

Forms of Muscles
Wide functional variation in terms of size and shape are defined according to the job done. The size of the functional component, the muscle fibre, varies from being 0.004 of an inch up to 12 inches in length. To put the diameter of a muscle fibre into context, consider that a fibre is typically ten times smaller than a human hair. Diameter, length, and arrangement of fascicles (bundles of fibres) will vary from muscle to muscle: fine bundles in precision muscles, coarse ones in power muscles. Fascicles may be parallel, oblique or spiral according to the position of attachments.

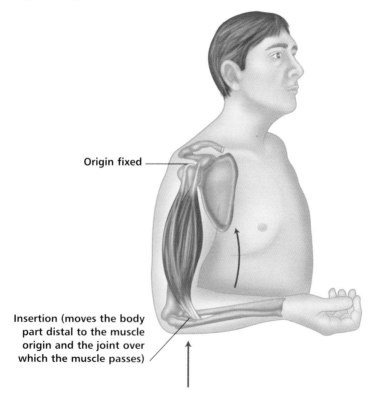

Origin fixed

Insertion (moves the body
part distal to the muscle
origin and the joint over
which the muscle passes)

Figure 2.12: Muscle working with origin fixed and insertion moving.

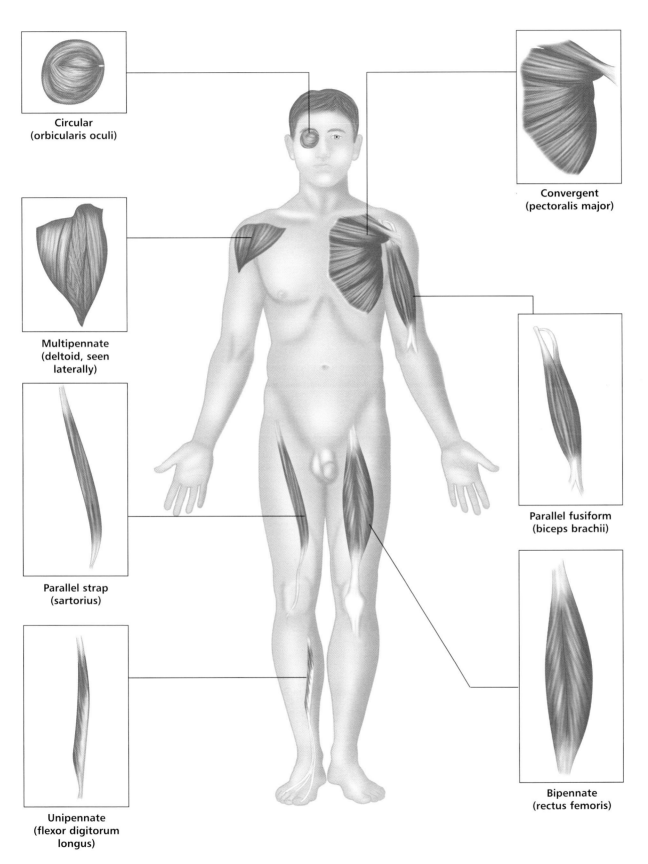

Circular
(orbicularis oculi)

Convergent
(pectoralis major)

Multipennate
(deltoid, seen
laterally)

Parallel fusiform
(biceps brachii)

Parallel strap
(sartorius)

Bipennate
(rectus femoris)

Unipennate
(flexor digitorum
longus)

Figure 2.13: Muscle shapes.

Variations (Shapes) and Explanations

The simplest is the *strap muscle*. This variation has a fleshy, wide attachment at each end. We can make this long and narrow, so long as the maximum length of the muscle fibre is not exceeded. If it is, we need fibres in parallel, with tendinous insertions between groups. The range of contraction depends on the length of a muscle but its power depends on how many fibres it contains. Strap muscles have a good range but low power: to get more power the muscle becomes fusiform, i.e. three-dimensional. This often transforms the flat attachment into a tendon with a circular cross section. The muscle fibres are often concentrated at one end, but will work just as well if they are digastric (i.e. have two bellies). Another way to increase power is to produce more heads, in effect two or three or four muscles pulling the same tendon.

Having more than one head results in muscle fibres pulling obliquely on the tendon. This can often balance out, but in a unipennate muscle, where fibres insert all along one side of a tendon the resultant force is the result of two vectors: sideways force is cancelled out in a *bipennate* or *multipennate* arrangement. Multipennates are common compound muscles with a short range but with lots of power.

Spiralized muscles not only pull the attachments together when they contract but try to untwist. A similar twisting is sometimes arranged by wrapping the course of a muscle around a bone. Good examples are levator scapulae and psoas major.

Action of Muscles

Muscles do not suddenly jump from a state of relaxation to one of contraction. At any given time functional units (motor units, groups of fibres of various size) will be contracting, some inhibiting and some in stasis; the end result provides muscle tone or a state of readiness. If the proportions doing each stay constant, so will muscle tone, although individual units will cycle. When an individual fibre contracts, it tends to approximate its ends, but whether or not this results in contraction depends on the force generated and the forces opposing the contraction. The net result for the whole muscle may be contraction, inhibition or stasis. A muscle trying to initiate contraction is opposed by:

1. Passive internal resistance of muscle.

2. Passive internal resistance of articular tissues.

3. Opposing muscles (inhibition).

4. Opposing soft tissues.

5. Inertia of whatever it is trying to move.

6. Load.

7. Gravity.

If the force generated exceeds the sum of all the above, the limb is accelerated from rest: once moving, a smaller force will keep it moving. A muscle doing this is referred to as the *prime mover* or *agonist*.

Antagonists can slow or stop the movement. When both groups act together nothing moves, or the movement is moderated or controlled. If the movement is abolished the real result is that the joint across which the muscles act will be stabilized. This cannot be done exclusively by close packing or gravity. Movement is always opposed or aided by gravity, and this is used wherever possible. The action of a prime mover often exerts a little unwanted movement. For example the flexion of the fingers by long flexors also flexes the wrists; this is opposed by wrist extensors.

It is easy to see that inhibited muscles cannot provide the decelerating force needed to avoid excessive end range of movement resulting in micro trauma. In a simple arrangement of two bones joined by a synergy of muscles, the pull of the muscles can be resolved into:

a. Swing. Tending to move the mobile bone.

b. Shunt. Compressing the joint.

c. Spin. Rotating the mobile bone.

Moving the attachments of the muscles varies the relative size of each component. The largest swing is best for initiating movement – spurt muscle. A large shunt will allow a mobile bone to be loaded by compressing the joint, and a large spin can be used for prime movement or as a synergistic "soaker-up" of unwanted rotation.

A *lever* is a rigid bar moving about a fixed point (*fulcrum*). More specifically, a lever consists of an *effort force*, *resistance force*, *rigid bar* and a *fulcrum*. The effort in a lever is a force applied to the lever in a specific direction and will cause movement in the lever if not balanced by an opposing force. The resistance in a lever is the force that opposes the effort force. The fulcrum in a lever is the support around which the lever pivots. Levers are classified according to the position of the fulcrum, resistance (load), and effort relative to each other. The combination of these relative locations results in first-class, second-class, and third-class levers.

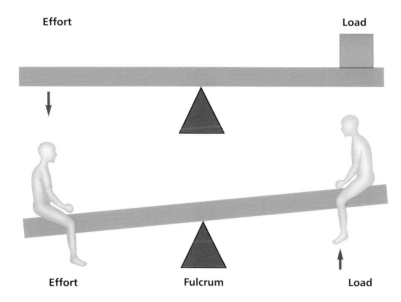

Figure 2.14: First-class lever (EFR): The Effort (E) and Resistance (R) are located on opposite sides of the fulcrum. Examples of a first-class lever include the jaws of life, seesaws, and crowbars.

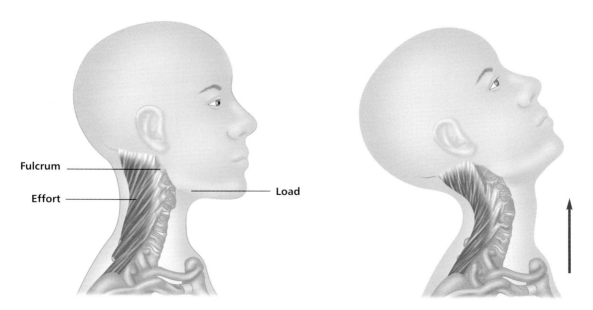

Figure 2.15: Second-class lever (FRE): The Effort (E) and the Resistance (R) are located on the same side of the fulcrum and the Resistance (R) is between the fulcrum and Effort (E). An example of a second-class lever is a wheelbarrow.

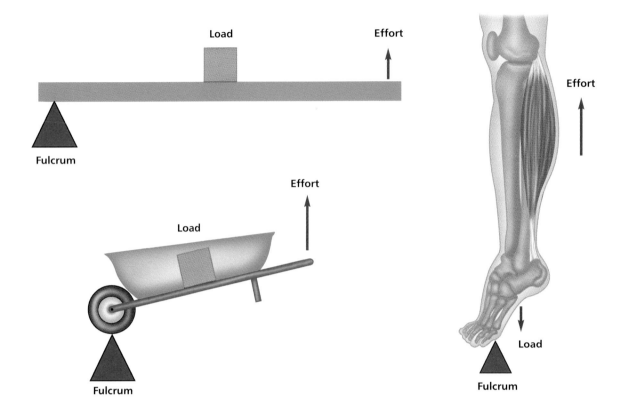

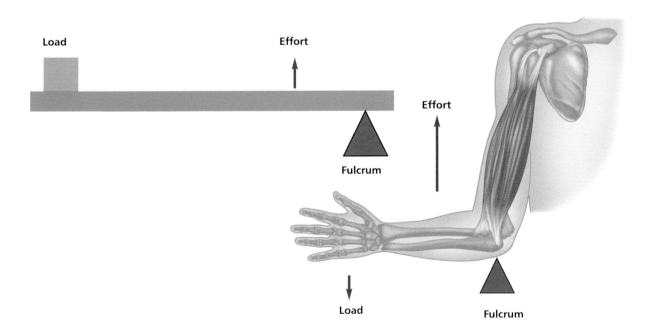

Figure 2.16: Third-class lever (FER): The Effort (E) and Resistance (R) are located on the same side of the fulcrum, but the Effort (E) acts between the fulcrum and the Resistance (R). Examples of a third-class lever include a shovel. A large effort gains speed of motion in this type of lever. It is the most common lever type in the human body.

Exercise Physiology: Theories and Proof

Theories

In the world of science there are many theories. The concept of evolution by natural selection, conceived by Charles Darwin, is a theory. Relativity described by Albert Einstein is a theory. The view that the earth orbits the sun, and not the other way around, is also a theory. Atomic theory is the notion that atoms exist. Each of these theories is an explanation that has been confirmed to such a degree, by observation and experiment, that we accept them as fact.

Understanding theories of muscle physiology will provide you with the foundation to understanding the various techniques used in NMT and their therapeutic outcomes. Of course we must continue to be aware of the future outcomes of quality academic research and be prepared to change our views whilst continuing to challenge our beliefs.

Proof

Newspaper and magazines articles often use headlines that are attention seeking with catch phrases such as "dramatic proof". With further reading and investigation it becomes obvious, all too often, that it is generally neither. The word "proof" has been a stick many have used with which to beat other less 'academic' therapies. Many claim that their therapy has been 'proven' to work. Shown to work, or demonstrated to have positive therapeutic outcomes is very different from proving. If academic research could definitely prove anything, cigarette companies would have been put out of business many years ago.

Cigarette companies used medical research to "prove" that smoking reduced the risk of contracting specific cancers. When the small list of such cancers is compared to the enormous list of smoking induced cancers, one appreciates the difference and can come to an informed opinion based on the current facts.

Therapies including NMT should be science-based. However, I caution all therapists to avoid the word "proven" and instead use softer terms such as "research supports", or "research has demonstrated". Research takes many shapes and sizes. One must consider what is being investigated and how it is being investigated. Is it quantitive or qualitative? How many people are included in the study, and how were these people recruited? All of these factors, and others, provide reliability and validity to a study. Empirical research focuses on data that has been collected, summarized, and analyzed. The conclusions drawn and the recommendations made in such studies can be no better than the data on which they are based. For example, if the instruments used to collect the data are not quality instruments, the data will be simply inaccurate. As more and more data is collected supporting the therapeutic effects of massage and various neuromuscular techniques, care is needed to ensure we do not beat other less academically supported therapies with the "proof" stick. Care is needed when choosing the vocabulary to describe the research supporting our therapy. Avoid the word "proof", "proven" or "proved". Not even Darwin could prove anything 100%.

Titin and the Sliding Filament Theory

In 1954 Huxley and Hanson proposed the *sliding filament theory*. The structural unit of muscles, the *sarcomere*, had been understood to consist of two interdigitating filament systems, which slide past each other when a muscle shortens. These special proteins were identified as being one thin and one thick protein filament. This description is the most widely used in medical and exercise science texts, even today.

Credit must be given to Huxley and Hanson all those years ago when they noted that removing the actin and myosin protein filaments did not lead to a collapse of the sarcomere. The presence of some third protein was proposed but their size and proximity to the other filaments made firm conclusions regarding their disposition and function, difficult to reach.

Over the years many descriptions have been used to describe the function of these filaments including S-filaments, gap filaments, T-filaments, core-filaments, and so on. In 1977 a new myofibrillar protein was identified and later in 1999 it was given the name *titin*. It appears that titin is the third most abundant protein of striated muscle, accounting for about 11% of the combined muscle protein content. Titin proteins cover a half sarcomere from the Z-line to the M-line.

I mention this, in that it is important to recognize that we are still learning about the architecture of sarcomeres. Of course that is why we still say the sliding filament theory, as it is the best theory we have to explain how muscles contract.

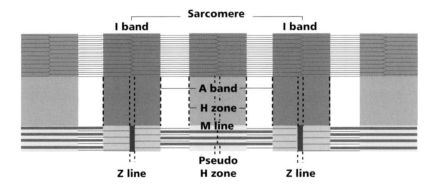

Figure 2.17: The myofilaments in a sarcomere. A sarcomere is bounded at both ends by the Z line.

Muscle Anatomy: Only One Muscle in the Human Body

This section is of the utmost importance in providing essential science related to the structure and workings of muscle fibres. Without this knowledge it is not possible to understand and appreciate the anatomy of trigger points. The following explanations are offered in a simplified science-based language yet offer a fresh view on the topic of anatomy. This view is one of connectiveness, a unified body, one muscle with 657 individual fascial bags or compartments.

Skeletal muscle attaches to and is continuous with the outer covering of bone, a connective tissue called *periosteum*. Skeletal muscle is squeezed by the fascia into individual bags. These fascial bags contain the central part of the muscle, called the *gastor* or *belly*, and the more condensed portions either end are called the *tendon*. This in effect means there is only one muscle in the human body. One continuous muscle with its associated fascia. This fascia raises and falls as it meanders throughout the body embracing the osseous tissue with its more solid component, the *periosteum*. Muscle tissue spirals and twists as it makes its way from origin to insertion. Muscle fibres are not arranged in straight lines but rather in spiral and diagonal patterns.

Not all tendons are thick cord-like structures: some are flat thin and/or thick tissues called *aponeuroses*. A good example of an aponeurosis is the thick tendon and fascia of the lower back known as the thoraco-lumbar fascia. The outer covering of muscle is called the *epimysium*, a tissue that encapsulates the entire muscle.

Each muscle contains subunits or bundles known as *fascicles*. Fascicles are, in turn, surrounded and separated by a connective tissue called *perimysium*. Fascicles come in various shapes and sizes. Each fascicle contains numerous numbers of individual muscle fibres or cells. Each individual muscle cell or fibre is separated from its neighbour by a connective tissue called *endomysium*.

The space between muscle fibres is called the *critical fibre distance* and should be maintained for normal healthy muscle function. When muscles are injured or dehydrated, this space can become compromised. The distance between the fibres reduces and the fibres become adhered.

Each individual muscle fibre has an outer covering or membrane called the *sarcolemma*. It is important to note that the sarcolemma maintains a membrane potential allowing impulses to travel along the muscle cell similar to nerves. Of course the main function of impulses in muscles is to generate or inhibit contractions. A muscle never relaxes. A typical muscle fibre is about one tenth the diameter of a human hair yet it can support 1000 times its own weight. Muscle names sometimes provide us with essential information regarding the muscles own individual features. Muscles received their names for many different reasons, such as:

Size Gluteus maximus (largest), gluteus minimus (smallest).
Position Tibialis anterior (in front (of the tibia)), tibialis posterior (behind (the tibia)).
Shape Deltoid (shaped like a triangle).
Number of tendons Biceps brachii (two-headed), triceps brachii (three-headed).
Fibre direction Rectus abdominis (rectus refers to straight).
Action Extensor digitorum (extend).

Now let's discuss the structure of the muscle cell. This will provide you with the necessary technical information to grasp how a muscle contracts and provide the foundation for understanding trigger point etiology.

Structure of a Muscle Cell

Muscle cells contain long protein strings called *myofibrils*. Each myofibril runs the length of a fibre. If a fibre is four inches long then the protein myofibrils making up that fibre will also be four inches long. Contained inside each myofibril are protein molecules called *myofilaments*. Each myofibril contains these special protein molecules within small-room like structures called *sarcomeres*. It is inside these sarcomeres that contractions take place. The special relationship between the various molecules contained within these sarcomeres causes a shortening, pulling the walls of each sarcomere closer together.

The outer covering of individual muscle cells, the *sarcolemma*, is designed with special holes and openings in it. These holes lead to tubes known as *transverse tubules* or *T tubules*. Similar in ways to microscopic blood vessels, these specialized tubes cover the myofibrils. T tubules function to conduct impulses originating on the surface of the sarcolemma into the muscle cell, specifically to the *sarcoplasmic reticulum (SR)*.

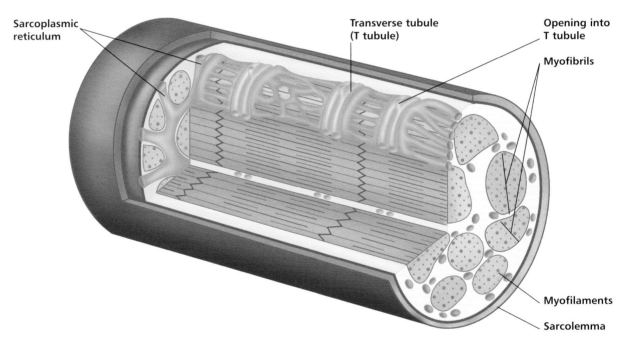

Figure 2.18: Structure of a muscle cell.

The Theory of Sliding (or Gliding) Filaments: Essential Information for Understanding the Formation of Trigger Points

The sliding filament theory is now internationally accepted as the basic mechanism for muscle contractions. The hollow sarcoplasmic reticulum functions to store calcium ions that are constantly being pumped into the sarcoplasmic reticulum from the cytoplasm of the cell. When muscle fibres are not contracted, a high concentration of calcium is located in the SR and low concentrations exist within the sarcoplasm.

Special calcium gates remain closed blocking calcium from escaping and moving into the sarcoplasm. When an impulse travels along the membrane of the SR these calcium gates open allowing a flood of calcium ions to rush out of the SR and into the sarcoplasm of the sarcomere where the myofilaments are located. This is a key step in the normal sequence leading to muscle contractions.

Myofibrils are composed of three types of myofilaments; *myosin* the thick protein, *actin* the thin protein, and *titin* the sticky protein. These myofilaments are arranged in a very precise pattern. The thick myofilaments are surrounded by six thin myofilaments while the titin proteins act as tails to anchor the myosin to the Z line. The thin actin myofilaments can be seen above and below each thick myofilament (see figure 2.17). In reality they spiral around the thick proteins in a snake-like fashion.

Within each sarcomere the myofilaments overlap similar to placing the bristles of two yard brushes into each other. When viewed under a microscope, the ends of a sarcomere appear lighter than the centre. This is because the thick myofilaments are situated in the centre while the thin myofilaments are located towards the ends. The name striated muscle was used for this reason. I-band is the name given to the light areas, while the dark areas are called A-bands. Near the centre of the I-band is a thin dark line known as the Z-line or Z-disk. The Z-line is where sarcomeres come together and the thin myofilaments of adjacent sarcomeres overlap slightly.

The thick myofilament called myosin (made up of two protein strands wrapping around each other) has a core or body with heads that project out like the head of a golf stick (two heads actually). These are called *myosin cross-bridges* (or -heads). These bridges or heads have a number of important facilities including:

1. ATP binding sites.

2. Actin binding sites.

3. A hinge allows a swivelling action so that the head can move the thin proteins resulting in a contraction.

Note the spherical shape of the long chains of actin molecules (also called G actins). The thin protein actin is constructed of two chains spiralling around each other. A smaller associated protein called *tropomyosin* in turn coils around the actin as shown. Another protein called *troponin* attaches itself at specific intervals to the tropomyosin. As these proteins are connected to each other, once the troponin moves, it in turn will pull the attached tropomyosin with it.

Here is the important point. Tropomyosin covers the binding sites on actin and when they are pulled away by the movement of those little proteins, troponin, the sites become free for the cross-heads (or -bridges) of the thick myosin to attach to and pull. This is how a muscle contracts.

What Makes the Troponin Move?

Understanding the sequence of events leading to a muscle contraction will provide you with a simple step-by-step picture of how a muscle fibre contracts. So far I have discussed the structure of muscle and described some of the key players. Now we must look at the chemical neurophysiology. I will keep it simple while at the same time I want to challenge you and advance your understanding. This will hopefully change the way you think about muscles.

Contractions: Pulling it all Together

When muscles are working normally, they require a nerve impulse (an action potential). This is the very first (or last) step leading to a contraction. This nerve impulse will travel along the sarcolemma and into the T tubules. From there the nerve impulse will travel to the sarcoplasmic recticulum leading to the active opening of calcium gates allowing calcium to diffuse into the sarcomere where the myofilaments are located.

Calcium now binds itself to the troponin molecule altering the shape of the protein causing it to move, thereby moving the attached tropomyosin. Now that the tropomyosin has moved, the myosin binding sites become free permitting the myosin heads to attach to and pull the actin. As the heads contact the actin, the myosin cross-bridges hinge and swivel pulling the myofilament actin, similar to a team in a 'tug of war'.

The pulling action occurs in a synchronized manner, some myosin heads attaching while others disassociate, but a collective effort leads to a concentric contraction. Should the pulling action be overcome by the external force or when a person consciously allows the muscle to be overcome, this leads to a lengthening of the muscle while it is pulling on the myofilaments. This is known as an *eccentric contraction*. Remember this means that muscles can only pull, they cannot push.

Of course, for muscles to work effectively energy is required and this is supplied by the breakdown of *adenosine triphosphate* (ATP). As long as calcium remains in the presence of the myofilaments, the sarcomeres will remain shortened. Under normal circumstances when the nerve impulse stops, the membrane of the sarcoplasmic reticulum is no longer permeable to calcium and the calcium gates now act in reverse allowing the calcium to escape from the sarcomere back into the sarcoplasmic recticulum. As the calcium disassociates with the troponin, it now pulls the tropomyosin back into its resting place covering the myosin binding sites. Tropomyosin now, once more, blocks the cross-bridges from touching the thin actin protein inhibiting a contraction from taking place. From this description of muscle contraction you can see that calcium is the 'key' that turns on a contraction, or for that matter turns it off.

If for some reason calcium ions cannot escape from the sarcomere, the myofilaments will remain shortened. It may require more energy to rectify this situation than to maintain it and so the muscle fibre remains short thereby increasing tension (i.e. a contracture). The seven steps of *cross-bridge cycling* are:

1. The influx of calcium, triggering the exposure of binding sites on actin.

2. The binding of myosin to actin.

3. The power stroke of the cross-bridges that causes the sliding or gliding of the thin filaments.

4. The binding of ATP to the cross-bridges, which results in the cross-bridge disconnecting from actin.

5. The hydrolysis of ATP, which leads to the re-energising and repositioning of the cross-bridge.

6. The transportation of calcium ions back into the terminal cisternae via the sarcoplasmic reticulum.

7. The provision of an action potential (this could be step 1 or 7).

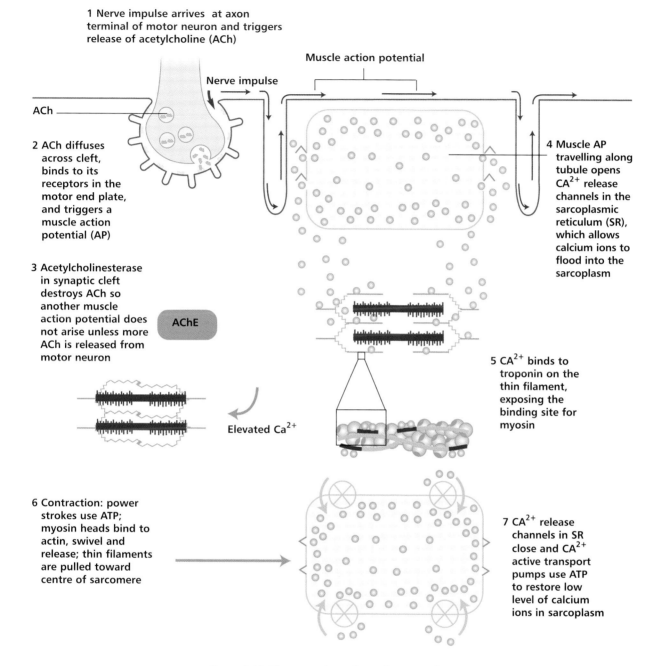

1 Nerve impulse arrives at axon terminal of motor neuron and triggers release of acetylcholine (ACh)

Muscle action potential

Nerve impulse

ACh

2 ACh diffuses across cleft, binds to its receptors in the motor end plate, and triggers a muscle action potential (AP)

3 Acetylcholinesterase in synaptic cleft destroys ACh so another muscle action potential does not arise unless more ACh is released from motor neuron

AChE

Elevated Ca^{2+}

4 Muscle AP travelling along tubule opens CA^{2+} release channels in the sarcoplasmic reticulum (SR), which allows calcium ions to flood into the sarcoplasm

5 CA^{2+} binds to troponin on the thin filament, exposing the binding site for myosin

6 Contraction: power strokes use ATP; myosin heads bind to actin, swivel and release; thin filaments are pulled toward centre of sarcomere

7 CA^{2+} release channels in SR close and CA^{2+} active transport pumps use ATP to restore low level of calcium ions in sarcoplasm

Figure 2.19: The seven steps of muscle contraction.

Exercise Science: Energy and ATP

Energy is not so much created or destroyed but is in fact converted from one form to another. It takes different forms such as light, heat, electrical, magnetic, and chemical. Animals from the lowly worm to humans all convert chemical energy from the food we eat to mechanical energy for work. When we do this we produce energy, but we also produce by-products including carbon dioxide, water, and heat. In fact, of the energy we produce only twenty per cent results in work or movement, with the remaining eighty per cent being released as heat. Just like humans, all animals use one exclusive chemical energy source for the production of this energy to run, walk, jump, digest food or have a thought. That chemical fuel is called adenosine triphosphate (ATP). It has to be produced and stored in all cells of the body. Only a small amount of ATP can be stored in the cells. When muscle cells contract, ATP is broken down into *adenosine diphosphate* (ADP) and one phosphate. Before ATP is broken down it consists of adenosine attached to ribose and three inorganic phosphates. The word *ribose* refers to a compound that is a building block of the backbone chains in nucleic acids. It is classified as a monosaccharide.

Muscle Fatigue

As ATP supplies begin to diminish, as they would if muscles are being used over an extended period of time or a short time of high intensity, myosin heads remain bound to actin and can no longer swivel. If calcium cannot escape from the sarcomere, the fibre can remain in a short state even though no nerve impulse is being received. This can lead to muscle spasm or at the micro level to tight muscle fibres. As muscles produce energy for high intensity activity through anaerobic metabolic pathways, the end result involves the production of lactates and inorganic phosphates. Lactic acid is often described as a waste product. This is not the case. As lactic acid builds in the muscle, being produced faster than it can be removed, this offers a feedback mechanism whereby the innervation of muscles diminishes and contractions can no longer be sustained. Finally, the individual would have to stop and catch their breath. If this important feedback mechanism did not exist the individual would most likely keep up the high intense activity resulting in a strain or a possible heart attack. An additional, and perhaps a more potent source of inhibition is the build up of inorganic phosphates as a consequence of the breakdown of ATP to ADP. Equine physiology takes advantage of adenosine diphosphates in a unique way. As ATP breaks down to ADP, one ADP gives up one of its two phosphates to another ADP thereby making ATP and *adenosine monophosphate*.

Motor Units

A motor unit is the combination of a motor nerve and all the muscle fibres that it connects to or innervates. When a nerve impulse travels the length of a nerve cell along its axon, all the muscle fibres attached to that nerve contract. A motor unit can have as few as three muscle cells or many thousands. This large variety of motor units provides muscles with the ability to perform precise or coarse muscle control. It also allows muscles to recruit increased numbers of fibres when needed depending on the required effort. This is known as *gradual increments of contraction* (GIC). It takes fewer motor units (and therefore fewer muscle fibres) to lift a 5kg weight compared to a 15kg weight. If we contracted all the fibres we have in a muscle every time we contracted that muscle we would not be able to distinguish between the effort required to lift a pencil compared to the effort needed to lift a telephone.

Muscular Tone

Muscular tone refers to the basic and constant ongoing contraction or muscular activity in the muscles, a state of "readiness" or preparedness. It can be understood as a baseline or background level of innervation. It is what helps to keep us upright or to give us "lift." Tone may be normal, too low, or too high. When muscular tone is too high (hypertonic), muscles can appear somewhat stiff and do not move in a smooth and natural way. A basic muscle tone that is too low or too high is one of the components of motor skills. Our view is to recognize and identify the hypertonic muscles and their inhibited (and therefore hypotonic) antagonist.

Gross Motor Skills

Gross motor skills refer to the ability of individuals to carry out activities that require large muscles or groups of muscles. Muscles or groups of muscles should act in a coordinated fashion to accomplish a movement or a series of movements. Examples of gross motor tasks are walking, running, throwing, and jumping. Posture is a very important element to consider in assessing gross motor skills. Adequate posture may make all the difference between being able or not able to execute a movement.

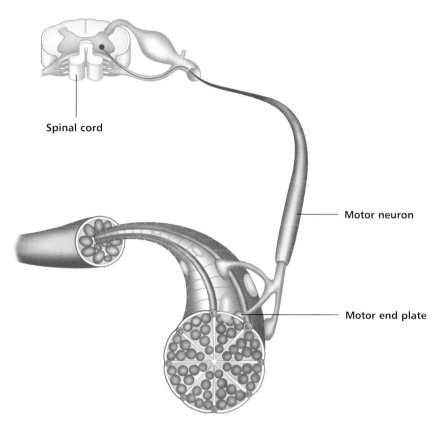

Spinal cord

Motor neuron

Motor end plate

Figure 2.20: A motor unit of a skeletal muscle.

Fine or Precise Motor Skills

Fine or precise motor skills consist of movements of small muscles that act in an organized and subtle fashion to accomplish more difficult and delicate tasks, e.g. the hands, feet, and muscles of the head (as in the tongue, lips, and facial muscles). Fine or precise motor skills are the basis of coordination, which begins with transferring from hand to hand crossing the midline when aged about six months. Examples of fine motor activities are writing, sewing, drawing, imitating subtle facial gestures, pronouncing words (coordination of soft palate, tongue, lips), blowing bubbles, and kissing. Many individuals, particularly children, who have difficulties in their fine or precise motor skills, also have difficulties in the articulation of sounds or words.

Trigger Points: Assessment and Treatment

3

Trigger Point (TrP) Formation Theories

Shoulder Anatomy, Arthrokinematics, and TrP Considerations

What is *Proprioception*?

Stages of Learning

Trigger Points (TrPs)

In this text, I refer to trigger points exclusively as hyperirritable localized spots (sarcomeres) found in taut bands within muscles. These spots are painful to touch and can provide referred pain, or a change in sensation distally or proximally, that is often recognized as the patient's primary complaint (numbness, itch, burning, pain, or coldness). Trigger points (latent or active) mimic everything from headaches to toothaches. Autonomic responses to trigger points include excessive sweating and salivation, goose pimples (*pilomotor reflex response*) or redness on the skin at the site of the Trp. For example, trigger points located in the paraspinal muscles can lead to hair loss in the associated dermatome. To date, trigger points are considered to be as a result of endplate dysfunction.

Such dysfunction results in a shortening of several sarcomeres (approximately 100 per trigger point) creating a palpable nodule in the muscle. Muscles can develop dozens of trigger points. Trigger points form at the centre of the muscle fibre, creating a taut band either side of the trigger point. Knowledge is needed regarding the arrangement of the fibres and number of muscle gastors, or bellies, in any given muscle. *Contracture* is when a sarcomere (or several sarcomeres) is shortened without the input of a nerve stimulus.

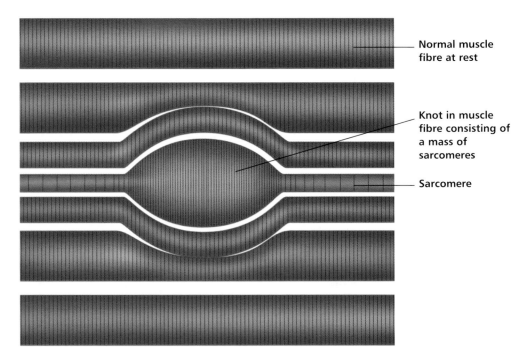

Figure 3.1: A trigger point showing 100 shortened sarcomeres without nerve stimulus and associated taut band (also called a contracture).

For example, rectus abdominis contains several gastors (four or more on both sides) and can potentially contain trigger points in each. All trigger points have the potential to refer pain. When a trigger point is created within the pain referral zone of another muscle, it is called a *satellite trigger point*. *Active trigger points* will refer a pain that the patient will recognize. *Latent trigger points* will refer pain but it will not be a recognized pain. Nevertheless, it may contribute 15%, 20%, or 30% plus of the patient's primary pain. Reducing pain by only 5% will be much appreciated by all patients.

Trigger Point (TrP) Formation Theories

Research and clinical experience has improved our knowledge to the why and how trigger points form and their mechanisms of referral (see Travel, J. & Simons, D. (1999), and Chaitow, L. & DeLany, J. (2002)). The following theoretical platform concerning the mechanisms of TrP formation and referral is based on sound physiology.

A dysfunctional endplate activity occurs, commonly associated with a strain such as unaccustomed physical activity or other soft tissue insult. Stored calcium is released at the site; acetylcholine (ACh) is released through calcium charged gates at the synapse, leading to an abundant and constant presence of this neurotransmitter.

Resultant ischemia develops and creates an oxygen/nutrient deficit accompanied by a local energy crisis. Energy (ATP) is needed in order to remove the excessive calcium. ATP availability is decreased by the ensuing tissue tightness. This in turn restricts local blood supply. The persistent high calcium levels maintain ACh release. A vicious cycle results.

ACh transmission causes the actin and myosin elements of myofibrils to slide into a shortened position, resulting in the formation of contractures (involuntary, without action potential). Removal of excessive calcium requires more energy than sustaining a contracture, so the contracture remains.

The contracture is sustained by the chemistry at the innervation site, not by action potentials. These are to be differentiated from contractions (voluntary with action potentials) and spasms (involuntary with action potentials). The actin/myosin filaments slide into a fully shortened position (a weakened state) in the immediate area around the motor endplate (positioned at the centre of the fibre). As the sarcomeres shorten, a contracture *nodule* forms, a palpable characteristic of a TrP. The remainder of the sarcomeres either side of this nodule within that fibre are lengthened, thereby creating a palpable taut band, another common TrP characteristic. Other characteristics are spot tenderness of a nodule in the taut band, and patient's recognition of pain or sensation by applying pressure on the tender nodule.

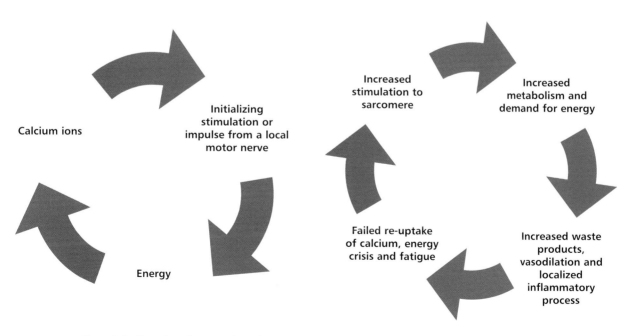

Figure 3.2: Flow chart for nerve impulse to cause muscle contraction.

Figure 3.3: Vicious cycle for trigger point physiology.

Additionally, there may be:

1. Visual/tactile evidence of local twitch response (LTR);

2. Imaging of an LTR may be induced by needle penetration of the tender nodule;

3. Pain or altered sensation in the target zone associated with that TrP when provoked;

4. EMG demonstration of spontaneous electrical activity (SEA) in the nidus (nucleus) of the TrP;

5. Painful limit to full stretch and reduced range of motion;

6. Muscle housing the TrP may test as weak;

7. Altered cutaneous humidity (dry or moist), temperature (cool or hot) or texture (rough);

8. A 'jump sign' or exclamation by patient due to extreme tenderness of palpated tissues including central (CTrP) and attachment (ATrP) trigger points.

Central Trigger Points

The previous description of a centrally located nodule describes a *central trigger point* (CTrP) that usually forms in the centre of a fibre's belly and is most likely associated with motor endplate activity. The CTrP is therefore defined as a palpable nodule at the centre of a taut band of fibres, which, when properly provoked, will refer pain, tingling, numbness, itching or a variety of other sensations. This associated referral pattern is referred to as a *target zone*. The target zone is usually located distally to the TrP, although it can be more central or, more rarely, can be within the local tissue where the TrP is housed.

Attachment trigger points (ATrPs) form where fibres merge into tendons or at periosteal insertions. Although ATrPs are not directly the result of endplate dysfunction (like the CTrPs), they are presumed to be indirectly a result of the CTrP since they develop at the attachment sites (periosteal, myotendinous) of the shortened contractured bands associated with a CTrP. ATrPs form at attachment sites where muscular tension provokes inflammation, fibrosis, and eventually, deposition of calcium.

As noted, central trigger points are located in the centre of muscle fibres while attachment trigger points form at the myotendinous junction or the periosteal attachment. This classification of trigger points will greatly influence the therapeutic application.

Satellite Trigger Points

Trigger points can also develop within the pain referral zone of active or parent TrPs. When such TrPs develop we refer to them as *satellite trigger points*, or *baby TrPs*. It is important when treating TrPs to treat all the muscles that refer pain within the target zone. If treatment is not having the desired result, immediate referral to the patient's general practitioner is advised. Trigger points in even small muscles can be the cause of extreme, debilitating pain. A recent study by Hsieh, Y-L. et al. (2007) provides evidence that dry needling evoked inactivation of a primary (key) MTrP situated in its zone of pain referral. This supports the concept that activity in a primary MTrP leads to the development of activity in satellite MTrPs and the suggested spinal cord mechanism responsible for this phenomenon.

Work Environment Considerations

Repetitive strains can result from manual working activity. Appropriate posture and correct arthrokinematics (or biomechanics) are essential for avoiding undue muscle stiffness and resulting compensations that can easily lead to the formation of myofascial trigger points. Sitting, in itself, places harmful forces and compressions without the added stress that working at a computer station can place on the neck, forearms, wrist and lower back. The height of the working desk and the relationship to the positioning of the computer relevant to eye level and neck flexion or extension is pivotal.

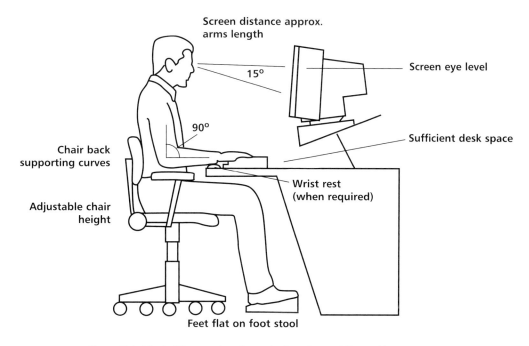

Figure 3.4: Ideal sitting posture for reducing stress while working.

Dietary Influences

Adequate quantities of minerals and vitamins are essential for healthy muscles and tissues. Many patients presenting with chronic pain are found to be deficient in a number of vitamins and minerals. Vitamin B_1, B_6, and B_{12} along with vitamin C and folic acid are important in the war on pain. Calcium, magnesium, iron, and potassium are critically important also. All too often people are confused as to why they are deficient in these important minerals and vitamins as they will report they eat well and have normal dietary habits when compared to other family members. The problem may not be their diet but rather their personal health choices such as smoking, drinking alcohol or caffeine. Smoking, for example, annihilates vitamin C while oral contraceptives affect vitamin B_6 levels. Antacid medication can leave many individuals with the symptoms of chronic fatigue. Even signing their signature becomes an effort.

Patients with vitamin and/or mineral deficiencies may report: feeling unusually cold, bouts of diarrhea, restless leg syndrome, headaches, disturbed sleep, and trigger point pain. Other symptoms include feeling fatigued, muscle cramping, and depression. Metabolic disorders should be ruled out particularly thyroid problems and hypoglycemia. Referral is recommended. Summary of types of trigger points:

Active Produces a pain recognized by the patient as their primary complaint and is active when the patient is at rest.
Latent Produces pain when palpated. This pain may not be recognized as the primary pain.
Primary Forms in response to trauma or insult.
Key Responsible for activating satellite trigger points.
Satellite Activated by key trigger points in its kinetic chain area of referral.
Central Located near the centre of the gastor or muscle fibres.
Attachment Located in the tendon of a muscle.

Contraindications to Trigger Point Therapy

1. Open wounds or broken skin should be avoided.

2. Malignancies. Should a patient state they have a malignancy, their GP or specialist must give written permission before any treatment can be given.

3. Aneurysm.

4. Haematomas. These should never be pressed, massaged or stretched.

5. Arteriosclerosis. Due to the risk of blood clot formation, GP or medical specialist approval must be provided in writing. Information regarding all medications should be provided.

6. Osteoporosis. This is particularly serious if using dry needle techniques due to risk of fenestrations (small holes that occur in bones such as the scapula through which the needle could contact the lungs if care is not taken).

Visceral pain has a temporal evolution, and in its early stages can be insidious and difficult to identify. Due to the low density of sensory innervation of viscera and the extensive divergence of visceral input within the central nervous system (CNS), what is called *true visceral pain* is a vague, diffuse, and poorly defined sensation regardless of the specific internal organ of origin. It is usually perceived in the midline at the level of the lower sternum or upper abdomen. Whether the origin is from the heart, oesophagus, stomach, duodenum, gallbladder, or pancreas, visceral pain in the early phase is perceived in this same general area.

Additional stimuli such as local compression applied to this area fail to worsen the pain. True visceral pain can easily be overlooked. This is due in part to the fact that the patient cannot clearly describe the pain. It is often described as a vague sense of discomfort, malaise, or oppression. It is typically associated with marked autonomic phenomena, such as pallor, profuse sweating, nausea, vomiting, changes in blood pressure and heart rate, gastrointestinal disturbances (e.g. diarrhea), and changes in body temperature. Strong emotional reactions are commonly present that include anxiety, anguish, and sometimes even a sense of impending death. Sometimes visceral pathology may manifest principally through vegetative and emotional reactions, with minimal pain and discomfort. A typical example is painless myocardial infarction, which may produce a sense of gastric fullness, heaviness, pressure, squeezing, or choking.

As a general rule, in these early stages, the intensity of visceral pain bears no relationship to the extent of the internal injury. Visceral pain should always be suspected when your patient presents with vague midline sensations of malaise. This is even further compounded when the patient is elderly.

As visceral pain continues to progress (minutes to hours) it may refer to dermatomes whose innervations enter the spinal cord at the same level as the visceral organ involved. This can be misinterpreted by the brain as joint, muscular or nerve pain manifesting itself as sharp, localized, deep somatic pain. For example liver pathology can lead to referred pain in the right upper shoulder. Peripheral nerve pathology such as irritation of the C7–C8 spinal nerves presents as pain in the fourth and fifth fingers (ulnar nerve). This type of pain can be accompanied by hyperalgesia (increased sensitivity, pain on light stimulation) or hypoalgesia (decreased sensitivity, numbness).

Detailed questioning of your patient is required to clarify their compliance and level of discomfort. During this stage (i.e. assessment) the NMT must determine the characteristics of the pain, the pathways of pain radiation or referral, its form and dependency from active, active resisted or passive movements. Feedback from the patient concerning neurological signs, skin sensitivity, pain and referral plus other symptoms including heat, cold, tingling, itch, mood swings are all vital ammunition in the war on pain. This information will ensure you refer the patient to the appropriate medical practitioner. If you are in any doubt at all refer to the patient's GP who will respect you for your professional approach and concern for your patient's health and wellbeing.

Once your patient returns to you they must supply a letter from their GP or medical specialist to state NMT is appropriate in this specific case and pathology is not suspected or has been ruled out. NMT's do not diagnose pathologies. That said, for many patients, the NMT may be the first foot soldiers they meet on the front line in their war against pain. As time can be such a crucial factor in pathology, referral without delay is always in the patient's best interests. As an example, here is an examination of the shoulder for trigger point activity.

Shoulder Anatomy, Arthrokinematics, and TrP Considerations

The glenohumeral (GH), scapulothoracic, suprahumeral, acromioclavicular, sternoclavicular and acromioclavicular articulations are the key joints (both true and false) affecting the shoulder. Structures that are anterior and medial to the glenohumeral joint include the biceps brachii and musculo-tendinous units including the pectoralis major, pectoralis minor, and subclavius. They also include the bony coracoid process.

Intra-articular structures include the supraspinatus and infraspinatus muscles, the labrum, capsule, bursa, and ligaments. Posterior structures include the scapula and the rotator cuff (SITS) and scapular stabilizing muscles, which include the triceps brachii, rhomboids, serratus anterior, trapezius, and levator scapula.

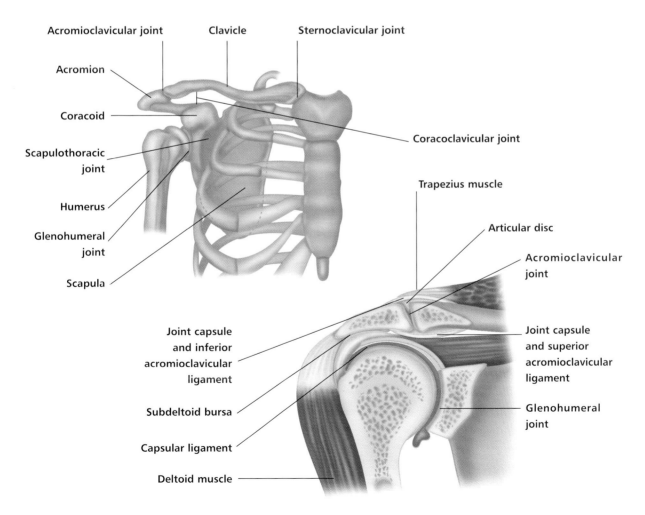

Figure 3.5: The anatomy of key articulations of the shoulder.

Depending on the patient's presentation, the assessment can be expanded to examine the cervical and upper thoracic spine, the brachial plexus and its branches, the sternoclavicular joint, and muscles such as the paraspinals and scalenes.

It is essential to utilize neuromuscular thumb or finger techniques to assess skin, muscle tone, and size, as well as monitoring and comparing pulses such as brachial and radial pulses. Trigger points housed in these muscles can squeeze both blood vessels and nerves leading to loss of sensation or hyper-sensations including burning, tingling, itching, and others. Trigger points can lead to a retardation of blood supply and cause cramping or swelling. Such body parts often feel cold. Long-term implications of reduced blood supply can lead to serious pathological disorders.

If the SITS muscles are not performing their role in drawing the head of the humerus into the glenoid during any action, similar to abduction of the humerus, it is possible to envisage a slipping posterior-inferior or anterior-inferior of the humeral head. This will result in a subluxation or in the more serious case a dislocation of the glenohumeral joint. This change in joint positioning and arthrokinematics is the basis for the formation of *functional trigger points* (FTPs). FTPs will evolve to provide tension or stiffness within the joint facility and likely in the most inhibited musculo-tendinous structures. This stiffness or tension is offered as a protective facility for short-term intervention. Unfortunately, these trigger points can become the source of unrelenting pain and reduced range of motion.

In frozen shoulder conditions, it is regularly noted that the pectoralis major is spastic, drawing the humerus into the side of the body and internally rotating the humerus in the GHJ. This has the effect of closing down blood supply to the GH region and providing the foundations for a sequence of events that compound the frozen shoulder syndrome. Upper trapezius will be short and overcontractured and the scapula will not demonstrate normal scapulohumeral rhythm.

General Rules for the Treatment of Trigger Points

1. Treat the most severe trigger points (TrPs).

2. Treat trigger points that are most medial and superior before those that are distal (inferior) and more lateral.

3. Treat those areas that have a cluster of trigger points as a priority.

4. When a muscle has several trigger points, initially treat the ones located in the centre of the gastor (muscle belly) or muscle fibres.

5. Only treat between three to five muscles in any one treatment in the earliest stages of treatment intervention.

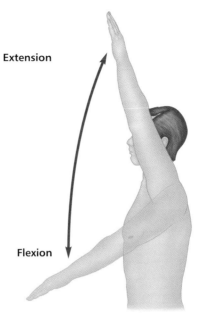

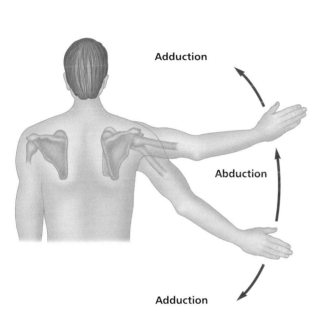

Figure 3.7: **Abduction:** Movement of a bone away from the midline of the body, or the midline of a limb.
Adduction: Movement of a bone towards the midline of the body, or the midline of a limb.

Figure 3.6: **Extension:** To straighten or bend backward away from the foetal position.
Flexion: Bending to decrease the angle between bones at a joint. From the anatomical position, flexion is usually forward, except at the knee joint where it is backward. The way to remember this is that flexion is always toward the foetal position.

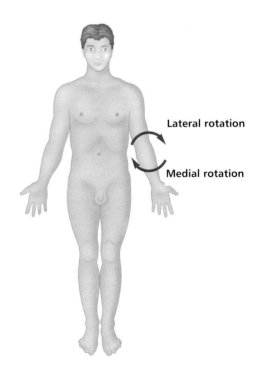

Figure 3.8: **Lateral rotation:** To turn out, away from the midline.
Medial rotation: To turn in towards the midline.

Shoulder Biomechanics (Arthrokinematics)

The glenohumeral articulation is exceptional due to its unique degree of mobility throughout the range of motion (i.e. three degrees of freedom). A) Flexion-extension, B) Abduction-adduction, C) Medial-lateral rotation.

Stability is maintained in the shoulder joint by the glenohumeral ligamental complex, the compressive forces of the rotator cuff, the glenoid labrum, negative intra-articular pressure and normal scapular kinematics as part of the scapulohumeral rhythm. The scapula moves in coordination with the moving humerus so that the centre of rotation of the joint remains within a *safe zone*. Trigger points can affect correct glenohumeral positioning. Coordinated muscle activity will reduce maximum concavity compression. Scapular retraction allows for full cocking ensuring an efficient and explosive forward acceleration of the arm. Scapular protraction allows for maintenance of proper glenohumeral positioning and facilitation of deceleration in follow-through.

The coupled motion of the arm and scapula provides dynamic stability for the glenohumeral joint in the various positions encountered in activity. It is easy to see how trigger points can interfere with this force couple action. Latent trigger points have been shown to interfere with this finely-tuned mechanism resulting in muscles firing out of their normal and appropriate neurological sequence.

Acromial elevation, necessary to prevent rotator cuff impingement, may be disrupted by fatigue of the serratus anterior, lower trapezius and the rotator cuff muscles due to TrP formation or loss of fascial integrity (e.g. spiral chain). The scapula therefore forms an important link in the kinetic chain mechanism in which large forces are generated in the proximal segments (legs, hips, and trunk) and transferred through the scapula into the shoulder and ultimately to the arm and hand (i.e. upper sleeve) for execution of some movement. Maintaining a stable *scapular platform*, in conjunction with core neuromuscular efficiency, allows for the most appropriate shoulder function.

Evaluation of the Shoulder

A thorough history is important and should include the mechanism of injury, location of pain, identity of trigger points, position of the arm when pain occurs, relieving and aggravating factors, activity modifications, prior injuries to the shoulder and kinetic chain structures, treatment update, sport or functional demands, and a general medical history. If there is a risk of dislocation, fracture, or serious pathology present, no special tests are required and the patient should be referred without delay.

As stated earlier, the proximal structures of the kinetic chain (legs, hips, and trunk) and the scapula are very much connected with shoulder function and should also be evaluated. Leg/trunk strength can be screened with one-legged stability tests. Such tests could include the one-legged stance, the one-legged squat, and the simple lunge test. Things to look out for are *Trendelenberg's sign* (dropping of the contralateral hip), knee valgus, pelvic rotation, increased lumbar lordosis, and forward lean. In general, these signs suggest weakness of the core lumbo-pelvic-hip muscles, which are the muscles of the abdomen and diaphragm, back, pelvis, and superior portion of the lower limb.

Thoracic and cervical posture should be assessed for thoracic scoliosis or excessive kyphosis and excessive cervical lordosis. Look for tenderness and trigger points by palpating on the spinous processes, paraspinals, levator scapulae, vertebral scapular border, rotator cuff muscles, serratus anterior, coracoid process, pectoralis minor, and biceps brachii tendon.

Supraspinatus strength can be assessed by resisted abduction in the scapular plane. Infraspinatus strength can be tested by resisted external rotation with the elbow at 90 degrees and the arm by the side. Both these muscles should be tested with the scapula retracted to eliminate the appearance of muscular weakness that can result from a protracted position, which does not allow the scapula to provide a stable base for muscle action. Subscapularis strength can be tested by internally rotating the shoulder and pressing the hand into the gastor, by internally rotating the shoulder and lifting the hand off the back against resistance, and by doing an uppercut manoeuvre against resistance.

Shoulder range of motion should be examined in flexion, abduction, and internal/external rotation at 0 degrees and 90 degrees. This test should be repeated with the therapist offering compression from both sides to the sacroiliac joint (*assisted force closure*). If the patient's pain reduces by at least 70% with increased range of motion when the test is repeated, the therapist can assume that the patient has reduced core stability. A medical exercise program to address this neuromuscular inefficiency should be put in place. Particular attention should be paid to determine the presence of *Glenohumeral Internal Rotation Deficit* (GIRD), which is associated with labral and rotator cuff injury.

An assessment of GIRD can be done by comparing side-to-side differences in internal rotation, measured using a goniometer with the scapula stabilized and the shoulder abducted to 90 degrees and then internally rotated to the point of tightness.

Abnormalities of winging, translation, and rotation are best assessed at rest and during shoulder abduction or flexion. Muscle weakness causing scapular dyskinesis is often seen as a hitch or jump, seen more in the descending phase of arm movement. This may be due to latent trigger points in associated muscles and can often be a red flag for lack of sacroiliac force closure and reduced core stability.

Based on the position, the dyskinetic pattern can be grouped into one of three visual positions that can help to identify involved kinetic chains.

1. In type 1 (lower trapezius weakness), the inferomedial border is prominent.

2. In type 2 (serratus anterior weakness), the medial border is prominent.

3. In type 3 (upper trapezius weakness), the superomedial border is prominent.

Dyskinesis is often present in more than one plane and it is more important to identify the presence or absence of dyskinetic patterns. A whole body kinetic chain perspective is required.

Arm abduction that elicits painful crepitus over the superomedial or inferomedial borders is suggestive of scapulothoracic bursitis, although trigger points must be ruled out as the true source of the symptoms. A treatment plan involving vigourous cryotherapy is recommended. Cold therapy should only be applied for 6–10 minutes several times a day but especially in the morning and last thing at night.

The *scapular assistance test* evaluates local scapular and acromial involvement in subacromial impingement. To perform this manoeuvre in patients with signs of impingement, the superior border is stabilized and then the inferomedial border is assisted to facilitate upward rotation, posterior tilt, and external rotation of the scapula during elevation of the arm. This procedure simulates the force couple activity of the serratus anterior and lower trapezius muscles. Elimination or reduction of impingement symptoms indicates that these muscles should be a focus of local rehabilitation.

The *scapular retraction test* involves stabilizing the scapula in a retracted position on the thorax. This position provides a stable base of origin for the rotator cuff muscles and will often facilitate an improvement in supraspinatus strength. It may also decrease pain related to internal impingement due to scapular and glenoid involvement as the glenoid has been removed from the excessively protracted position that causes impingement. These findings indicate that subsequent NMT rehabilitation should focus on endurance strength of the rhomboids and trapezius.

Quantitative measurement of scapular stabilizer strength can be achieved by means of a *lateral scapular slide test*. This test compares the position of the scapula in the injured and non-injured sides in relation to a fixed point in three different positions: arm at the side, hands on the hips with the fingers anterior and thumb posterior with about 10 degrees of shoulder extension, and arms at 90 degrees of elevation with maximal internal rotation of the glenohumeral joints.

In each position the distance between the inferior angle of the scapula and a fixed bony point on the spine is marked on each side. A side-to-side difference of at least 1.5 cm in any of these positions can be considered abnormal.

Glenoid labrum integrity can be clinically tested by palpating for tenderness along the anterior and posterior joint lines while moving the joint through its range of motion and by the following manoeuvres.

The anterior slide test is undertaken with the patient's hand on his or her hip, fingers anterior and thumb posterior, and the shoulder in about 10 degrees of extension. The examiner applies an upward force to the elbow while the patient resists this motion.

NMT Test 1

With the patient's shoulder flexed to 90 degrees and internally rotated, the examiner applies a downward force to the elbow while the patient resists this motion.

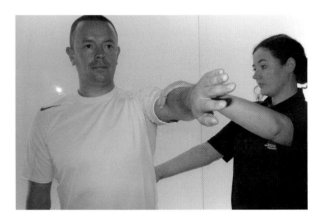

Figure 3.9: NMT test 1.

NMT Test 2

With the patient's elbow flexed, shoulder abducted to 90 degrees and externally rotated. The patient resists the examiner's attempt to extend the elbow.

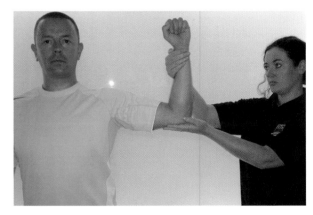

Figure 3.10: NMT test 2.

NMT Shear Test

Place the patient's shoulder into a 90-degree angle of abduction, then passively externally rotate and pull down. The examiner palpates the posterior joint line.

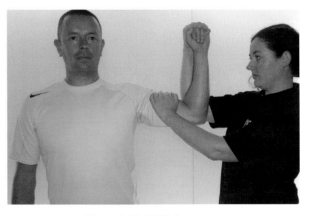

Figure 3.11: NMT shear test.

The NMT tests described are considered positive if there is a reproduction of pain. Glenohumeral instability should be assessed, by including an anterior and posterior drawer or compression test. Inferior instability is assessed using a sulcus test.

For all these tests, the scapula is first stabilized and the two sides compared. Then the arm is held and translated anteriorly for anterior instability and posteriorly for posterior instability. For the sulcus test, the arm is distracted inferiorly to create a sulcus (groove or furrow) between the acromion and the humerus. A test is considered positive if the translation generates pain and/or there is increased laxity in comparison with the other shoulder.

Medical exercise has been advocated to restore motor control to the upper and lower extremity. In the clinic, the term *balance* is often without clear definition. Details such as static and dynamic conditions, equilibrium, and biomechanical stress and strain must be considered. Efferent or motor response to sensory information results in activities affecting muscle tone, motor execution programs, cognitive somatic perceptions, and reflex joint stabilization.

Proprioceptors or mechanoreceptors are located in and surround each joint. They are composed of *Ruffini cells*, *Golgi tendon organs* (GTOs), *muscle spindles*, and *free nerve endings*. Each of these sense organs plays a different role by the type of information it sends to the central nervous system (CNS). These sense organs are found in the joint capsule, the muscle gastor, tendon, and retinaculum, as well as in the various ligaments supporting a joint. The ankle has the most mechanoreceptors followed by the hip and knee.

The relationship between proprioception and balance is important. The body uses three systems to keep itself upright against gravity. The vestibular system centred in the inner ear is the foundation of the balance mechanism. This mechanism is enhanced by input from vision. It is further assisted by information from the mechanoreceptors. Injury damages the mechanoreceptors. This damage will cause a diminished ability to know where the joint is in space and time and an inability to detect motion. This directly affects skilled movements and indirectly affects balance. Detecting this loss is important to the medical exercise rehabilitation process. Medical exercise rehabilitation for lower or upper extremity injuries should centre on proprioception, endurance, range of motion, strength, flexibility, power, and agility.

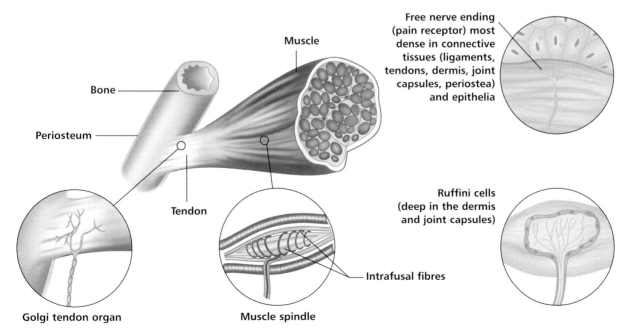

Figure 3.12: Anatomy of the muscle spindle, Golgi tendon organs, Ruffini cells, and free nerve endings.

What is *Proprioception*?

Proprioception is a specialized variation of sensory modality. It has been described as the perception of body awareness. It is a sense that people rely on daily, yet are frequently not aware of. More easily demonstrated than explained, proprioception is the unconscious awareness of where the various regions of the body are located in relation to each other at any given time.

I recommend both balance and proprioceptive training combined as an integral part of medical exercise to restore motor control. Proprioception and balance are separate entities yet intricately related. This is achieved through medical exercise programs.

Proprioception is the forerunner of appropriate balance and function. Balance can be described as the process by which we control the body's centre of mass with respect to the base of support, while either being static or moving. This can include the ability to maintain a position, the ability to voluntarily move, and the ability to react to a perturbation. The three components of balance are important in the maintenance of an upright posture. The three components are:

1. Static balance is an individual's ability to maintain a stable antigravity position at rest by maintaining the centre of mass within the available base of support.

2. Dynamic balance involves automatic postural responses to the disruption of the centre of mass position.

3. Reactive Postural Responses (RPR) are activated to recapture stability when an unexpected force displaces the centre of mass. RPR can be demonstrated by anyone closing their eyes and moving their leg around in a circle (i.e. circumduction).

Assuming proper proprioceptive function, at no time will the person lose awareness of where their leg actually is, even though it is not being detected by any of their other senses.

To fully comprehend proprioception and proprioceptive training (a keystone of medical exercise), one must appreciate that as you perform physical actions, the overall muscular activity, joint range of motion, and posture are all the products of sensory nerve activities received, coded, and acted on by the central nervous system (CNS). The CNS receives the information needed to control movements from three *subsystems* within the body:

1. The somatosensory system;

2. The vestibular system;

3. The visual system.

The somatosensory system contains nerves located in the skin, bones, musculo-tendinous junctions, and joints. The somatosensory system can detect touch, pressure, pain, and joint motion and position. In joints, the somatosensory system possesses both *quick-adapting* (QA) and *slow-adapting* (SA) *mechanoreceptors*, nerve endings that detect physical actions. Should a joint be stimulated continuously by pressure or motion, the QA mechanoreceptors decrease their signalling of the CNS, while the SA mechanoreceptors keep the CNS fired up.

Mechanoreceptor experts believe that the sensation of joint motion is mediated primarily by QA mechanoreceptors, with SA mechanoreceptors playing more of a role in telling the CNS about joint position and sensation. In the human knee joint, mechanoreceptors have been identified which respond specifically to joint acceleration and deceleration.

Human muscles contain mechanoreceptors which report to the CNS concerning muscle length and tension (i.e. spindles and GTOs) and which work with the joint QA and SA mechanoreceptors to give the brain and spinal cord comprehensive information concerning what is happening elsewhere in the body. Proprioception is referred to as the collection of sensations regarding joint movement (kinaesthesia) and joint position at any given time in space.

Sherrington first described the term *proprioception* in the early 1900s. Proprioception has been defined in many ways. Current thinking divides proprioception into two categories. The first category is the ability to know where a joint is in space and time. It is also the ability to reposition a joint to a previously experienced position either actively or passively.

The second category is called *kinesthetic awareness*. This is the ability to detect motion at a joint. These are two very important hallmarks of skilled movement. Proprioceptive information is transmitted to the spinal cord via afferent or sensory pathways. The information travels at 70 to 100 m/sec. This is much faster than pain signals, which travel at only 1 to 3 m/sec. This information contains details such as static and dynamic conditions, equilibrium, and biomechanical stress and strain. Efferent or motor response to sensory information results in activities affecting muscle tone, motor execution programs, cognitive somatic perceptions, and reflex joint stabilization.

Typically, ligament loading and rupture can occur in the 70 to 90 m/sec range while reflex arc reactions occur in the 40 to 80 m/sec range. Cortical response can take up to between 120 and 150 m/sec to be elicited after ligament loading. With this in mind it is important that any neuromuscular response delay is eliminated with medical exercise to reduce the risk of injury.

As we perform work against gravity, the body utilizes the three sub-systems to keep itself upright. The vestibular system, positioned in the inner ear, is the primary member of the balance mechanism. This mechanism is further enhanced by input from vision and further assisted by information from the mechanoreceptors. Injured tissues or joints cause a diminished ability to know where the joint is in time and space and an inability to detect motion. This directly affects skilled movements and indirectly affects balance. Special tests are required to detect this loss so that a graduated program of physical activities can be provided as part of the medical exercise rehabilitation process.

Three levels of the CNS are activated with this medical exercise rehabilitative balance based training. The spinal reflex is the simplest. It is used in reactive situations triggered by external stimuli. The response regulates muscle responses that are highly stereotyped. These activities are characterized by sudden alterations in joint position that require reflex muscle stabilization. In medical exercise we recommend the use of rhythmic stabilization activities as they stimulate the spinal reflex arc. Perturbation activities are also an excellent way to develop this facility. This can be done while the patient is balancing on one leg or two legs or while standing on an unstable surface.

The second level of the CNS to be activated by medical exercise balance training is at the brain-stem level, which is also triggered by external stimuli. The response is automatic. It is not as stereotypical and therefore can be impacted by medical exercise balance training.

Response time is within the 90 to 100 m/sec range and composed of coordinated movement patterns. Medical exercise balance training activities with and without visual input will enhance motor function on the brain-stem level. Neuromuscular balance activities at this level should be progressed from bilateral stance to unilateral stance, from eyes open to eyes closed, and from a stable base to an unstable base.

The third level of CNS that should be activated with medical exercise balance training is the cerebral cortex. This is the highest level of control where mechanoreceptor information interacts with, and influences, cognitive awareness and movement in which motor commands are initiated for voluntary movements. These activities take place in the 120 to 150+ m/sec range.

Training at the level of the cerebral cortex stimulates the conversion of conscious programming to unconscious programming—taking the conscious mind out of the activity. Examples of training at this level would include throwing a small ball to the patient while they are trying to balance on an unstable surface.

Medical exercise is used to offer a progressive program of functional physical activity that is critical for restoring the synergy and synchronicity of muscle firing patterns required for dynamic stability and fine motor control. The main objective of medical exercise is to return patients to their pre-injury activity level as quickly and as safely as possible.

NMT's achieve this by enhancing the dynamic muscular stabilization of the joint while increasing the cognitive appreciation of the respective joint in regard to both position and motion. This is achieved following appropriate intervention with neuromuscular therapy applications such as trigger point deactivation.

Medical exercises are designed to restore joint functional stability and enhance motor control skills. Program design must include a graduated manipulation of the environment in order to facilitate an appropriate response and make use of balance and proprioception. Control is provided over the joints that dominate the task in which plane the activity is taking place.

Restoring dynamic stability, an important component of functional movement, requires challenging the proprioceptive and balance systems. Dynamic stability allows for the control of abnormal joint translation during functional activities. Neuromuscular balance training through medical exercise is essential to enable the patient with upper extremity orthopaedic injury to return to physical activity.

Reestablishing neuromuscular control is a critical component of medical exercise in the rehabilitation of pathological joints. The objectives of the medical exercise activities are to integrate peripheral sensations relative to joint loads and process these signals into coordinated motor responses. This muscle activity serves to protect joint structures from excessive strain and provides a prophylactic mechanism to recurrent injury. Neuromuscular control activities as part of medical exercise are intended to complement rehabilitation protocols.

Elements crucial for reestablishing neuromuscular control and functional stability include: joint proprioception and kinesthesia, dynamic stability, preparatory and reactive muscle characteristics, conscious and unconscious functional motor patterns. Dynamic joint stabilization exercises additionally encourage preparatory agonist/antagonist co-activation. Efficient co-activation restores the force couples necessary to balance joint forces and increases joint congruency, thus reducing the loads imparted on to static structures.

Medical exercise focuses on stimulating the reflex pathways from articular, muscular, and tendinous receptors. Although preprogrammed muscle stiffness can enhance reflex latency, the objective is to induce joint perturbations that are not anticipated and will stimulate reflex stabilization. The last element requires preprogrammed adaptations to functionally specify motor patterns and joint loads.

Pathophysiology

Motor coordination is the product of a complex set of cognitive and physical processes, often taken for granted. Smooth, targeted, and accurate movements, gross and fine, necessitate the harmonious functioning of sensory input, central processing of this information in the brain and coordination with the higher executive cerebral functions (e.g. volition, motivation, motor planning of an activity), and finally, carrying out of a certain motor pattern. These elements must work in a coordinated and rapid way to enable the execution of complex movements with the different parts of the body.

Adequate realization of a motion or sequence of movements requires the convergence of numerous pathways and a central system in charge of integrating the information. The motor cortex, cerebellum, and vestibular system (providing input about directionality, gravity, motion) are all part of this central mechanism.

Proprioceptive information (i.e. sensation of where the body is in space and also the positions of the various limbs and parts of the body), visual input (i.e. where the body is in space and where it should go), and an adequate degree of alertness (i.e. the reticular formation activated to an optimal degree) are ingredients that provide information to the central nervous system. If one of these systems is not functioning adequately, the resulting planned movement may not be satisfactory or smooth and the risk of injury and formation of trigger points increases.

Medical exercise programs designed to comprehensively address proprioceptive aspects of the joint may protect against injury. Specific proprioceptive training can help to fine-tune the afferent-efferent arcs.

Medical exercise activities should include repetitive, consciously mediated movement sequences performed slowly and deliberately as well as sudden, externally applied perturbations of joint position to initiate reflex, subconscious muscle contraction. It is not possible to single out specific mechanoreceptors to train, but certain activities can enhance mechanoreceptor activation and therefore have an effect on the central nervous system pathway.

To improve the proprioceptive system in dynamic joint stability, a challenge is required. In injury, *pain free* should not be mistaken for *cured*. If the proprioceptive deficit is not addressed, complete rehabilitation will not have been accomplished. Correction of a damaged static restraint (e.g. surgical correction of mechanically disrupted tissue) may not maximize the afferent neuromuscular input needed to enhance dynamic joint stability. Mechanically stable joints are not necessarily functionally stable, especially in less constrained systems such as the shoulder.

These activities incorporate all of the available resources for stimulating peripheral afferents, muscle co-activation, reflex control, and motor programming. Emphasis should be placed on sports or life-specific techniques. With repetition and controlled intensity, muscle activity (preparatory and reactive) gradually progresses from conscious to unconscious motor control. The lower extremities function in a closed-chain manner during daily life activities, and sporting activities.

In the upper extremities, medical exercise application of graded, multidirectional manual resistance can provide proprioceptive feedback in a closed-chain fashion. Open-chain manual resistance exercises with rhythmic stabilization (rapid change in direction of applied pressure) are also considered proprioceptively enriched. In either case, resistance can be modified, depending on pain, as the patient progresses.

Integrating Local and Global Muscle Units

In European Neuromuscular Therapy, local muscles are identified as those muscles involved with providing support for joints in the form of *stabilization*. Such muscles are located throughout the body and are less involved with specific movement. Local muscles provide the stability and increased stiffness required to ensure safe and effective joint movement.

Global muscles are ultimately responsible for creating movement. Such muscles are larger in size and attach the pelvis to the costal bones, providing a link between the lower limbs and upper quarter. A muscle creates force when it contracts. This force in turn creates stiffness. Force creates joint torque supporting postures and creating movement.

There are times when the force will enhance joint stability while other times it will compromise stability. It all depends on the magnitude of the force and its comparative degree relative to all other muscle forces acting at the joint. In contrast, the role of muscle stiffness is always to provide stability.

A stiff muscle supports against perturbations in all planes. Stiffness at one joint supports the development of explosive power at another. Stiffness is also improved by positional techniques of the body segment linkage where one segment can be stiffened against another. When all muscles that act on a joint stiffen together, a *superior stiffness* occurs. The total stiffness provided at the joint by all the muscles contracting together will provide more stiffness than any one muscle could on its own. As an example let us look at the abdominal wall in creating *core stability*. Rectus abdominis, external and internal obliques, and transversus abdominis unite together as a unit to create this superior stiffness that is greater than the sum of each individual muscle. In the neck this superior stiffness is provided by the infra- and suprahyoids and the sternocleidomastoideus (SCM) during activities such as sit-ups. If the tongue is not placed in its physiological resting position behind the front teeth in the roof of the mouth, the hyoid muscles cannot contract to create the level of stiffness required to offer cervical joint support.

The SCM will contract even more to make up the stiffness deficit resulting in short SCM, forward head posture, rounded shoulders and full body kinetic chain implications. In higher intensity activities which demand greater core stability, all muscles must be activated. High performance in athletics requires rapid muscle activation and force development, together with equally rapid reduction of muscle force. Superior stiffness needs only to occur briefly in such cases, but if it needs to be brief, the motor control system must be highly tuned to ensure optimal superior stiffness.

Stages of Learning

The first stage of learning is the *cognitive stage*. This is the initial training stage and requires a high level of cognitive awareness regarding the patient. This is the time when the patient is improving the *perception* of the skill, understanding the task, and getting to know what it feels like.

For example, cognitive awareness is necessary in order to isolate the co-contraction of the transversus abdominis and multifidus without substitution of the global muscles (e.g. rectus abdominis, external and internal obliques, thoracic portion of erector spinae). The objective of the first stage is to train the specific isometric co-contraction of transversus abdominis with lumbar multifidus at low levels of maximal voluntary contraction including appropriate breathing, in weight bearing within a neutral lordosis. The NMT needs to provide instructions, visual cues, mental imagery, optimal body positions or postures, and various facilitation/feedback techniques to encourage the ideal response.

The second phase of motor learning is the *associative stage*. At this stage, the focus is on refining specific movement patterns that have been identified as faulty and/or pain provocative. The objective is to identify a small number of these movement patterns during examination so that during rehabilitation they can be broken down into component movements and performed for a number of repetitions. The patient is taken through these component movements whilst isolating the co-contraction of the local muscle system.

Initially, exercises are performed whilst maintaining the spine in a neutral lordotic posture and the patient subsequently progresses to normal spinal movement. At all times segmental control and pain control must be ensured. Some of the movement patterns identified during examination may include sit to stand, walking, lifting, bending, twisting, extending, and so on. The patient is prescribed independent exercises that focus on the movement components. These are performed on a daily basis with pain control emphasized. Physical activities are progressed as speed and complexity of the movement pattern is increased. In time, these movements should be performed in an efficient neuromuscular manner. The patient should also perform exercises like walking while maintaining correct postural alignment, low-level transversus abdominis and multifidus co-contraction, and appropriate breathing.

A key issue in pain control is focusing on *muscle control* (performing the co-contraction) during movement patterns throughout the day that a patient would typically anticipate resulting in lower back pain and instability. This is fundamental to ensure that the co-contraction during these movement patterns becomes automatic. This stage can last from between eight weeks to four months. Rehabilitation time depends on motivation and compliance of the patient along with intensity of practice. It also depends on the degree and nature of the pathology.

The third and final stage is the *autonomous stage* where the participant requires a low degree of attention for the correct performance of the motor task. This stage involves specific exercise intervention, whereby subjects can dynamically stabilize their spines appropriately in an automatic manner during the functional demands of daily living. Multiple studies show that changes to automatic patterns of muscle recruitment can be achieved. The key is a decrease in recurrence of symptoms and better functional outcome.

How to progress:

1. Independent activation of transversus abdominis and multifidus.

2. Independent co-activation of transversus abdominis and multifidus.

3. Improve precision.

4. Co-ordination of breathing (may include paradoxical breathing as a common problem needing correction).

5. Function: Simple to more difficult static tasks.

6. Function: Easy to difficult dynamic tasks.

7. Local and global co-activation.

8. Specific progressive functional retraining.

Kinetic Chain Anatomy and Patient Assessment

4

Prime Movers,
Stabilizers, and
the Kinetic Chain

Kinetic Chain
Anatomy

Looking at Muscle
Function

Patient Assessment

Laws of European
Neuromuscular
Therapy

Muscle Energy
Techniques

The Term 'Agonist'

The major theme of this chapter is that muscles do not work alone. Any muscle performing an action is providing a portion (or all) of its available muscle's fibres, while the arrangement allows it to provide a *line of pull* (i.e. directional force) to offer a given movement at a given joint. For example, muscles with fibres running vertically on the anterior side of the knee joints are agonists of extension. Conversely, muscles with a portion of their fibres running vertically on the posterior side of the knee are agonists of flexion.

That being said, the word *antagonist* is often used to describe a muscle that opposes a specific action. If a person contracts their biceps brachii concentrically (agonist) the triceps brachii must lengthen with inhibition to allow flexion at the elbow to occur (antagonist). This in my view does not describe an antagonistic relationship but one rather of partnership, of agreement. This finely-tuned partnership allows fluent movement and controlled acceleration and deceleration throughout range of movement (ROM) that protects muscles and joints, and ensures appropriate joint space. There are special movements that occur that require both an agonist and its antagonist to contract at the same time. This is known as a *co-contraction*.

Agonists, antagonists, synergists, stabilizers, and neutralizers must work effectively and synergistically to provide neuromuscular efficiency.

Prime Movers, Stabilizers, and the Kinetic Chain

Many soft tissue and myoskeletal injuries concerning the spine and extremities are caused or perpetuated by muscle imbalances and weakness in the core musculature. People with a weak core substitute primary muscles to compensate during dynamic functional movements. Popular machine-based exercise may be a significant contributing factor leading to overuse injuries as so many people overuse this type of equipment.

The core system is ultimately a system of stabilization. If it is not functioning optimally the result is neuromuscular substituting to utilize the strength, power, and neuromuscular control in the rest of the body. Unfortunately many individuals use exercise to develop strength and neuromuscular control in their prime movers neglecting core stabilization, or even worse, establishing ineffective kinetic chain patterns that prove stressful and lead to pain and injury. Understanding the kinetic chains will assist you in connecting pain in the head or neck to possible tension or spasm in muscles or fascia some distance away, even in the feet. By appreciating these relationships, you can carry out visual, structural, neuromuscular assessments to identify those tissues that are short, tight and spastic (possibly housing trigger points). Treating those structures first and providing a fascial release will provide the foundation for the possibility of a return to homeostasis and the introduction to functional movement challenges.

Stabilization

Analysis of movement will usually focus on the moving bone or segment. Focus must also be on the muscle forces that produce movement in that segment. Equal force is being exerted on the 'stable' part (or bone) known as the *origin*. When the biceps brachii exerts force on the radius, an equal force is also placed on the muscle's attachment to the scapula (coracoid process and glenoid fossa). In this example, the scapula does not move due to a stabilizing force offered by the muscles attaching to it.

When your vastus lateralis, medialis, intermedius, and rectus femoris exert force on your tibial tuberosity, your tibia will move. The stabilizing force in this example is gravity; the weight of your body would be too much for the muscles to move. When you perform a sit-up (on the floor) the abdominal muscles will pull the rib cage towards your pelvis. However an equal and opposite force is pulling on your pelvis yet it does not go into posterior pelvic tilt. Why? The pelvis will not posteriorly tilt due to forces generated by the hip flexors. Now think of what force will help to stabilize the lower extremities to which the hip flexors attach? All this time, what forces are acting on the vertebrae (think kinetic chain), all the way up to the base of the occiput? *Sharkey's Law of ROM* (lack of stability leads to tension which, in turn, leads to a loss of ROM).

Kinetic Chain Anatomy

The lumbo-pelvic-hip (LPH) complex musculature produces dynamic forces and stabilizes the kinetic chain during functional movements. Many of these deep pelvic muscles provide support to the pelvic viscera and help to maintain intra-abdominal pressure. More than 29 muscles attach to the core unilaterally. They are: rectus femoris, semitendinosus, semimembranosus, biceps femoris, psoas major/minor, iliacus, rectus abdominis, internal and external obliques, transversus abdominis, pyramidalis, quadratus lumborum, quadratus femoris, obturator internus and externus, gemellus superior and inferior, adductor longus, brevis, magnus, gracilis, pectineus, gluteus maximus, medius, minimus, tensor fasciae latae, erector spinae (iliocostalis, longissimus, spinalis), latissimus dorsi, multifidis, piriformis, levator ani, and coccygeus.

The primary function of the core's myofascial structures, including fascia and ligamentous chains, is to provide postural control by keeping the centre of gravity over our base of support during dynamic movements.

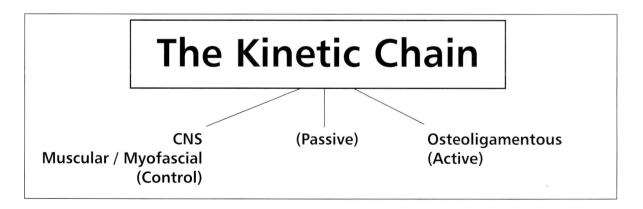

Myokinetic Chains and Sub-links

Primary neuromuscular strategies exist that coordinate muscular contraction in whole body stability and orientation. All of the body systems and structures work together to establish links that are ultimately interdependent of each other to form a *functional kinetic chain*. Within European Neuromuscular Therapy these strategies are known as the *spiral/oblique chain*, *lateral chain*, *posterior sagittal chain* and *anterior sagittal chain*. Several other secondary chains and/or links also co-exist, being both deep and superficial. These chains and links exist as one continuous facility through which forces are translated and dealt with through the periosteum out into the fascia and vice-versa linking toes to head and head to toes.

The Spiral (Oblique) Chain (S/OC)

The spiral (oblique) chain includes the external oblique, internal oblique (contra-lateral), adductors, iliotibial band, tibialis anterior, and peroneus longus/brevis. This chain can also include the following links: serratus anterior, ipsilateral rhomboids and contra-lateral splenius capitis).

The Lateral Chain (LC)

The lateral chain includes the peroneals, iliotibial band, tensor fasciae latae, the gluteals, external and internal obliques, ipsilateral adductors, quadratus lumborum (contra-lateral). The lateral chain may include the following links: intercostals, sternocleidomastoideus and splenius capitis/cervicis, scalenes).

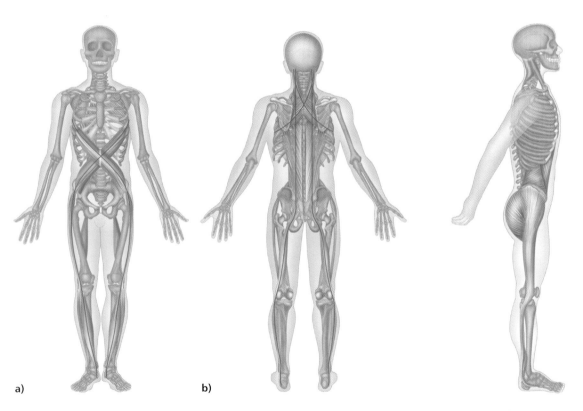

a)   b)

Figure 4.1: The spiral (oblique) chain (S/OC); a) anterior view, b) posterior view.

Figure 4.2:
The lateral chain (LC).

Posterior Sagittal Chain (PSC)

The posterior sagittal chain includes the thoraco-lumbar fascia and muscular links both above and below, offering movement and support to the joints of the periphery as well as to the spinal joints. At the mid-section, sub-links include the transversus abdominis and posterior fibres of the internal obliques. The pelvic floor muscles include pyramidalis, multifidi and lumbar portions of the longissimus, iliocostalis and the diaphragm, already described as the core. Of course this joint support system is also present at the glenohumeral and lumbo-pelvic-hip (LPH) complex.

A deep posterior or sagittal chain involves local, deep, segmentally related muscles providing stiffness to a motion segment or joint (Tonic Type II).

A superficial oblique posterior chain involves prime movers or more global muscles that are, as the name implies, predominantly superficial. These muscles are primarily phasic or Type I fibres with a high resistance to fatigue.

The posterior sagittal chain includes occipitofrontalis, erector spinae, thoraco-lumbar fascia, multifidus, sacrotuberous ligament, and biceps femoris (short head). This link can be continued to include the gastrocnemius and plantar fascia.

The posterior oblique links (POL) includes latissimus dorsi, contra-lateral gluteus maximus, thoraco-lumbar fascia. This chain can be continued to include the following links: iliotibial band, tibialis anterior, and the peroneals.

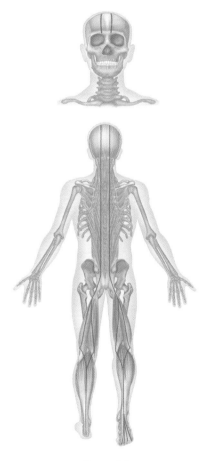

Figure 4.3:
The posterior sagittal chain (PSC).

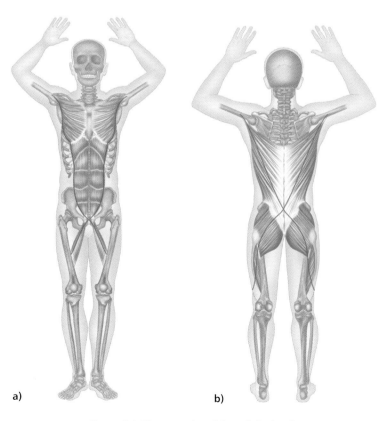

a)   b)

Figure 4.4: The posterior oblique links (POL);
a) anterior view, b) posterior view.

The Anterior Sagittal Chain (ASC)

The anterior sagittal chain includes the dorsal surface of the foot, tibial periosteum, rectus femoris (including articularis genu), AIIS (anterior inferior iliac spine), pubic tubercle, rectus abdominis, sternal periosteum, sternocleidomastoideus, and periosteum of the mastoid process.

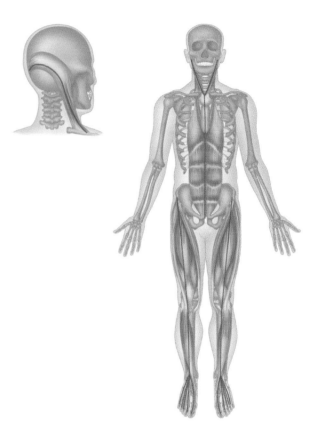

The Deep Anterior Chain (DAC)

The deep anterior chain includes the inner arch of the plantar surface (first cuneiform), tibialis posterior, medial tibial periosteum, adductors, linea aspera, ramus of the ischium and pubis, lesser trochanter, iliacus, anterior longitudinal ligament, psoas major, central tendon of diaphragm, mediastinum and pericardium, pleural fascia, prevertebralis fascia, fascia scalenes, longus capitis, hyoid and associated fascia, mandible, occiput, and galea aponeurotica.

Figure 4.5: The anterior sagittal chain (ASC).

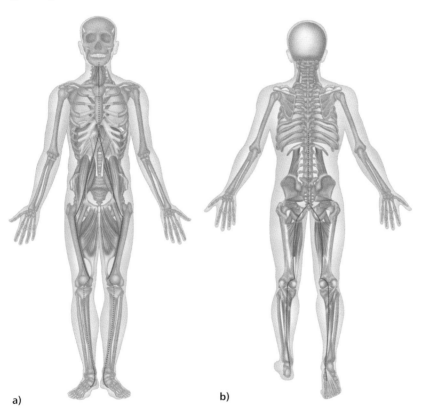

a)   b)

Figure 4.6: The deep anterior chain (DAC); a) anterior view, b) posterior view.

Looking at Muscle Function

Anatomically, muscles are wrapped into fascial bags containing the fibres in which contractions take place. Although the fibres are only located within the belly, or gastor, of a muscle the connective tissue, that is the fascia, continues on to become the tendon. It then continues on to become the outer covering of bone known as the *periosteum*. Periosteum continues along the shaft of a bone and will rise up to become a tendon of another muscle. This way of learning about muscles will, for many, be in stark contrast to the way medical students are encouraged to think of muscles.

Muscles may have anatomical individuality but have no functional individuality. In fact, there is only one muscle in the human body. This muscle is continuous from superior to inferior, anterior to posterior, side to side, birth to death. Muscle makes up about 35% of human body weight and 85% of body heat produced is from the muscles.

The fascia not only wraps up and covers the muscles but also the viscera and the skeleton (i.e. your bones). The fascial coverings wrapping up your organs and viscera are called the *subserous fascia*. The fascia just beneath your skin is called the *superficial fascia* (subcutaneous). It is one continuous chain of connective tissue throughout the body linking distant body parts to each other. From embryonic development, a system of interconnecting tubes including your arterial system and alimentary system combines with an interlocking system of fascial planes including the crural fascia, around the legs, merging at the inguinal ligament with the transversalis fascia surrounding the peritoneal cavity and continuing up to connect to the diaphragmatic fascia. On it continues to merge with the parietal pleura surrounding the lungs and continues its journey to merge with the cervical fascia on up from the neck onto and into the head.

The idea of compartmentalizing muscle function has led to the invention of machine-based exercises such as the back extension, leg extension, leg curl, and abdominal crunch.

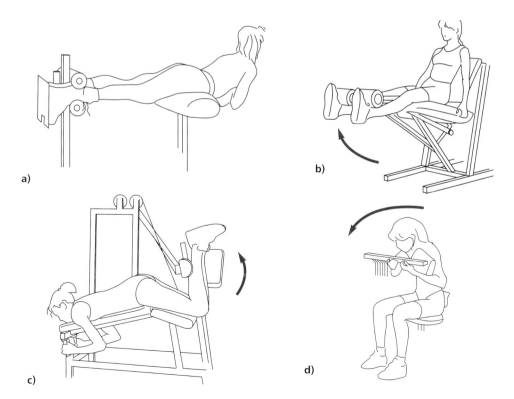

Figure 4.7: Machine-based exercises; a) back extension, b) leg extension, c) leg curl, d) abdominal crunch.

I want to encourage a shift in perspective from trying to isolate and improve strength in one muscle to improving multidirectional, multidimensional, neuromuscular efficiency (the firing patterns throughout the entire kinetic chain). It is important to recognize that the body does not contract only one muscle when performing a task but rather a number of muscles in specific sequence or concert. As muscles contract to accelerate, decelerate, stabilize, and neutralize, those forces generated are being facilitated along the continuous formed chains of myofascial tissue. A global view of human movement is required.

What is Form Closure?
Form closure addresses how the topography of the contacting surfaces of a joint and its ligaments contribute to stability and reduce or prevent shearing and excessive translation between the two joint surfaces when under load.

What is Force Closure?
Force closure addresses the forces necessary to control translation between two joint surfaces when under load. For example, at the sacroiliac joint, the force required for controlling shear is compression. The stabilizing muscles of the lower back and pelvis in conjunction with the fascia through the sacrotuberous ligament provide this compression. They include the transversus abdominis, multifidus, pelvic floor, and biceps femoris of the lower limb.

Let's first take a look at 'machine-based' exercise. Medical exercise incorporates machine-based exercise. However, if an individual does not integrate whole body *kinetic chain* functional exercises into their program, the risk of muscle dominance, neuromuscular inefficiency, adaptive postural changes and risk of injury may increase.

Machine-based exercise can promote neuromuscular inhibition resulting in the nervous system shutting down prime movers. To avoid this, a focus on stabilizing the core with functional or life specific physical activit, through the LPH complex is included.

How Does this Occur?
Firstly, machine-based exercises are usually *unidirectional* (i.e. in one direction) while all functional movements are *triplanar*, i.e. movement occurs in all possible planes. Triplanar movement requires acceleration, deceleration, and dynamic stabilization. A number of machine-based exercises have no functional relationship to how humans move or live. For example, you would never reach for an item in the way you move your arms while performing an abdominal crunch (see figure 4.7(d)).

Couple that with the fact that your trunk and hips are flexed while generating substantial forces, and one can visualize and appreciate how this repetitive action could promote poor motor patterns and poor posture, e.g. rounded shoulders. This however, does not mean that machine-based exercises are necessarily bad.

The central nervous system (CNS) recruits muscles in groups or synergies allowing movements to be organized in such a way as to reduce unwanted movements. The result is a smooth economical action. Over time and through a sequence of learning synergies, movement becomes more anatomical and fluent.

Understanding muscular synergies will enable you to appreciate functional anatomy and related biomechanics. The human body is ultimately designed to provide movement in an integrated and connected chain. Physical activities such as exercise and training should reflect this.

Muscle synergies or 'links' organize movement in a coordinated manner so as to minimize the amount of unwanted movement at a joint or joints. Once a motor pattern has been learned, the CNS will fine-tune and automate this alliance ensuring its fluency with time and practice. This is an example of the *law of facilitation*.

Example: A child eating an ice cream cone gets more ice cream on their face than in their mouth. Of course as they mature and grow so to does their nervous system. With practice and experience, they learn to accurately place the ice cream in their mouth. This requires timing, co-ordination, reaction time, balance, and a collective 'integration' of neural activity. Ice cream ending up on the face is not the required result and the child learns from augmented feedback known as *knowledge of results* and *knowledge of performance*. These relate specifically to the outcome of a performance and the quality of the overall movement sequence or plan. Of course, relearning to perform an action in a manner that does not stress the muscular, myofascial, articular, or neural system will require re-education.

Once a person has established a neuromuscular synergy specific to a task they will always perform that task utilizing the same muscles in the same sequence. Over time this may pre-dispose that individual to postural adaptations, inappropriate neural activity, muscular inhibition, joint stress and ultimately injury. In other words if a person learns to perform something incorrectly, they will always perform it incorrectly. Once the movement or posture is learned the neurological engram is established and muscles will be recruited in a specific sequence, the same sequence every time that person performs that task. Learning to do it correctly will feel odd and uncomfortable.

Atrophy
Atrophy could be defined as the progressive loss of muscle mass (or wasting), caused by the reduction in the size or number of muscle cells.

Hypertrophy
Hypertrophy involves the increase in both the size and diameter of muscle fibres. This occurs when quantities of the proteins that make up muscle fibres, including structures such as mitochondria, increase their size and number in the sarcomere.

General Adaptation Syndrome and Local Adaptation Syndrome
Changes at a local level will have an effect on the larger global picture. Changes are occurring all the time, moment to moment in the human body. Some changes lead to positive adaptations, whilst others create problems that have been termed, *bad gas*. The cumulative effect of a small number of local minor areas of stress can result in more global adaptations due to the demands being placed on a constant basis.

Inflammation
Inflammation is the body's reaction to tissue injury. Although it is often seen as something to be avoided, it plays a vital role in the repair and recovery of tissue injury. Inflammation is a protective facility that provides the first step in repair responding to burns, cuts, tears, and chemical irritation, as well as invasion by bacteria or viruses.

A potential problem exists in that the rate or level of inflammation is in direct proportion to the extent of trauma the tissue undergoes. When tissue damage occurs, a series of reactions take place, including the release of histamine and other irritable chemicals, e.g. kinins. This results in vasodilation at the injury site and an increase in permeability of the walls of the capillaries. This increase in blood flow results in a temperature increase and redness. Excess swelling results from changes in the capillary walls allowing blood plasma to escape into the interstitial fluid. This in turn increases the pressure within the affected tissue, irritating special pain receptors (nociceptors) resulting in pain. Pain and swelling will obviously have an effect on limiting range of motion, thus reducing the risk of further damage.

The tissue fills with plasma, and an increase in phagocytes and white blood cells is seen in the damaged tissue. Phagocytes engulf any damaged cellular debris cleaning the area and removing any foreign invaders that could cause infection. Specialized clotting agents stick together to reduce blood loss and seal any leaks. Now the tissue can begin regenerating new tissue. As is often the case, the body lays down additional collagen fibres as a specific adaptation to the original tissue damage. This is a protective mechanism to reduce the risk of injury reoccurring at the same site. However, although the initial collagen is organized along the axis of the muscle fibre arrangement, additional collagen is often unorganized, which leads to scar tissue. This is why movement in the earliest stages of injury recovery is so vital. Many people rest the injury for far too long and in the case of upper limb injuries, may avoid involving the limb in daily activities. This is detrimental and not only prolongs recovery, but can lead to increases in scar tissue and loss of range of motion.

A sequence of events following tissue injury usually includes muscular splinting or spasm. While the initial inflammation is an integral stage in correct healing, it does need to be controlled. The resulting protective spasm (and possible formation of trigger points) is the real culprit and needs to be addressed and returned to homeostasis before any additional exertion or physical activities are encouraged. Failure to address this spasm, coupled with the introduction of exercise, will only offer temporary relief. Once the physical activities stop, the patient usually finds that their problem returns. The *missing link* is to treat the spastic tissue first and then re-educate the muscles through graded functional physical challenges.

Patient Assessment

Before prescribing medical exercise, such as in a rehabilitative program, or performing any type of neuromuscular therapy, a complete and comprehensive patient assessment is called for. This is the time to carry out the kinetic chain postural assessment and take a detailed patient health history.

The cornerstone of any assessment must be to include a postural component. Of course motivational interviewing is essential to get to know your client or patient. There is little point in asking a patient to participate in water-based physical activities if they do not like being in water. It is vital to listen to your patients. Discover what they wish to achieve, their likes and dislikes, and their current daily tasks. This will allow both your client/patient and you to identify an appropriate, effective yet safe rehabilitative medical exercise program that fits their lifestyle. Realistic goals can be identified within an appropriate time frame.

A framework is required involving testing muscle for shortness, relative weakness, range of motion, neuromuscular reflexes, and postural (a)symmetry. Such deficiencies can be the cause of, or contributor to, pain and change in respiratory function. Nutritional and psychosocial influences should also be considered.

Muscles that shorten due to stress include: gastrocnemius, soleus, adductors, psoas major, tensor fasciae latae, rectus femoris, piriformis, quadratus lumborum, erector spinae, pectoralis major/minor, teres major, upper trapezius, levator scapulae, and sternocleidomastoideus.

Muscles that tend to be inhibited include: tibialis anterior/posterior, serratus anterior, vastus medialis oblique, middle/lower trapezius, articularis genu, rhomboids, transversus abdominis, teres minor, internal oblique, infraspinatus, multifidus, posterior deltoid, and the deep cervical muscles.

Ask your patient to shade in areas of pain, referral or changes in sensation on the silhouette. This will help you as a visual aid in determining what muscles may be housing trigger points responsible for or adding to the patient's complaint.

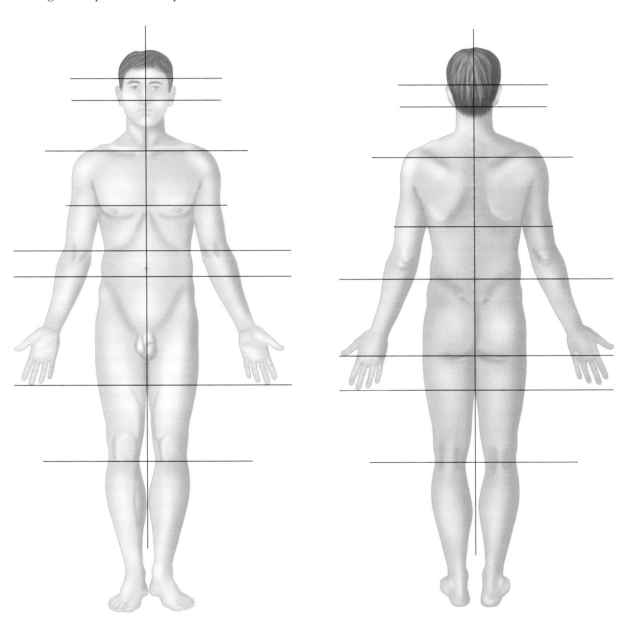

Figure 4.8: Body outlines on which patient should shade areas of pain, referral or changes in sensation.

Training Principles

Physical activities can provide both health and/or skill-related components of fitness. Our primary focus in rehabilitation is to provide the correct mix to offer improved joint health and neuromuscular efficiency. Consideration must be given to the following principles: progressive overload, specificity, reversibility, variation, and individual difference. Let's now look at these principles in more detail.

Progressive Overload

An appropriate physical activity is provided to produce optimal physical, physiological, and performance adaptations. A program of medical exercise will provide the effective and safe level of physical effort to ensure appropriate progressive adaptations. The components include the volume (number of repetitions and sets), intensity, contraction velocity, muscle action, recovery period, training frequency, plane of motion, exercise selection, and order of performance.

Specificity

Adaptations that occur due to physical activity are specific to the kinematic and kinetic demands placed on the person. The outcomes of the chosen activities will be specifically related to the motor unit synchronization, rate coding, motor unit involvement, and rate of force production (neuromuscular specificity). Choosing movements that mimic, or are related to, the patient's daily activities ensure improved movement patterns that are specific to their lives. This is known as **S**pecific **A**daptations to **I**mposed **D**emands or **SAID**.

Reversibility

This principle has two variations on the theme. The first variation refers to the loss of gained improvements and neuromuscular efficiency should the patient cease their involvement in physical activity. The second variation refers to reversing the status of damaged, weak, or dysfunctional tissues to homeostasis. Once successful rehabilitation has occurred, the focus of physical activity can be to maintain neuromuscular efficiency and provide the basis for a reduced risk of injury in the future.

Variation

Changes are required concerning the type of stimulus provided. Changes involving speed of movement (acceleration and deceleration) and stabilization within all planes of motion should be provided. Medical exercise should provide the patient with the multi-planar, multi-dimensional training necessary to ensure a progressive and systematic scale of physical activities.

Individual Difference

Designing a medical exercise program requires consideration of the patient's needs and realistic goals. Consideration therefore must be given to their age, medical, and health status (and history, including injuries), and gender. Look at the following sequence for progressing a program of physical activity:

- Set up the program with simple familiar movements and progress to more complex ones involving all three planes of motion.

- Begin with simple static challenges and progress to more dynamic movements.

- Move slowly at first then add speed.

- Provide tactile, visual, and verbal support to ensure effective and appropriate force couples.

- Low forces are appropriate for beginners rising to high forces.

- Start with one arm movement, and then progress to two arms.

- Begin with two leg movements and progress to one leg.
- Initiate with stable surface movements moving on to unstable surfaces.

- Once your client/patient loses form, the exercise is finished. Remember it is not about repetitions. It is quality not quantity.

- Ensure your patients avoid breath holding.

- Avoid static stretching, and encourage dynamic range of movement (DROM).

Step One

A health history questionnaire is required. If a client/patient has a history of blood pressure, coronary heart disease, or any other life-threatening chronic illness, he/she must get clearance, in writing, from their doctor. Certain medications can be of significant importance to the therapist or medical exercise specialist and the patient's doctor should be consulted for any special guidelines or contraindications. Learning about your patient's health history provides you with vital information to help you make the best-informed decisions regarding treatment strategies and appropriate physical activities and tasks. For example, low back pain can cause decreased neural control of stabilizing muscles to the lumbo-pelvic-hip (LPH) complex resulting in reduced stabilization of the vertebral column. Injuries to the lower limb, in particular the ankle, may decrease neural control of the gluteus maximus and medius muscles, while shoulder injury is related to neuromuscular retardation of the SITS muscles. Any letters or documents pertaining to your client/patient should be affixed to their file.

A Few Words on Client Records

Your clients' records are strictly private and confidential and they are, in effect, the property of your patient. You can only share their information with other professionals once your client has given you written permission to do so. All records must be secured under lock and key and must be retained for up to no less than seven years.

Step Two

Interview your patient regarding their reason for treatment. It is essential to get a clear picture of what the patient requires and to ascertain if those expectations are both within your scope of practice and realistic. At this stage the patient should shade in any areas of pain or heightened sensations on the silhouette provided. A red felt tip pen should be used for this purpose. This information can provide a visual impression of their experienced pain patterns or change in sensation. These may also provide a link to trigger point referral patterns.

Step Three

Postural assessment-kinematic chain evaluation begins the moment you meet your patient. Careful observation concerning your patient's movements, and during static posture, can provide valuable insights. You should observe the manner in which your patient walks. For example, do the arms swing evenly with a matched pace and rhythm or is one arm held short, or perhaps closer to the body? When standing still, do the arms hang down by the side with the hands semi-supinated and the little finger in line with the seam of their trousers? Observe the space between the line of the elbow and rib cage. Is more light seen through one side as opposed to the other?

Anatomical landmarks can be used to compare symmetry. Very small differences exist in all of us but significant differences can help identify short, spastic, or hypertonic tissues and assist in recognizing inhibited muscles. To help your patient avoid feeling self-conscious, the use of *distractions* can be helpful. Ask your patient to march on the spot for sixty seconds, and then repeat this with their eyes closed. On stopping, some patients have a tendency to pull their body up and suck their tummy in. Turning your patient around while their eyes are closed can result in a slight disorientation and often allows a more realistic image of their true posture to be witnessed. Global and local compensations may be identified standing 10 to 15 feet away from the patient.

Postural Considerations

Examples might include head tilt, forward head, rotated head, shoulder level difference, pro/retracted shoulder girdle, standing on one leg in preference to the other, locked knees, accentuated or flat spinal curves, scoliosis, level of the ends of fingers with arms hanging by the side, knee cap positioning, flat feet, or feet turned out/in.

Anterior Mid-sagittal Plane

The anterior mid-sagittal plane includes the nasal septum, sternum, belly button (umbilicus), and symphysis pubis.

Anterior Transverse Horizontal Plane

The anterior transverse horizontal plane includes the crown of the head, eyes, ears, acromion, ASIS, crest of ilium, crease of elbows, tip of fingers, patellae, head of fibula, and medial malleolus.

Coronal Plane

The coronal plane includes the auditory meatus, head of humerus, greater trochanter, head of fibula, lateral malleolus, and ASIS relative to PSIS.

Posterior Mid-sagittal Plane

The posterior mid-sagittal plane includes the occipital protuberance, spinal processes, sacral tubercles, and coccyx.

Posterior Transverse Horizontal Plane

The posterior transverse horizontal plane includes the acromioclavicular joints (AC), inferior angles of scapula, crest of ilium, PSIS, gluteal fold, creases of knee, and straight calcaneal tendon.

Two calibrated scales can be used side by side with the patient standing on the scales with one foot on each scale. Weight bearing should be bilaterally close to even, although a small differential is normal (optimal posture is being sought). Significant differences to look out for include:

- Is the head erect or leaning/turning to one side?

- Are both eyes level?

- Are both ears level (mastoid process)?

- Is the distance between the ear lobe and the acromion symmetrical bilaterally?

- Is the nose straight?

- Does the midline of the mandible track in a smooth and straight (vertical) line when opening and closing?

- Are the AC joints level?

- Is there any obvious internal /external rotation noted regarding the position of the arms?

- Is there a slight bend in the elbows?

- Are the fingertips level?

- Are the hands slightly pronated with the dorsal surfaces facing 45 degrees anteriorly?

- Are the fingers relaxed and slightly curved?

- Is the space between the arm and torso bilaterally symmetrical?

- Is the general appearance of the torso balanced?

- Are the rib cages bilaterally symmetrical?

- Is the distance between the inferior angle of the ribs and the iliac crest even on both sides?

- Is the ASIS level on both sides?

- Are the greater trochanters level with each other?

- Do the patellar bones look even, level, and symmetrical?

- Are the anterior fibular heads level?

- Are the malleoli even?

- Do the feet look turned in/out?

- Are the arches normal/high/fallen?

Step Four
Implementation of a NMT treatment plan based on stages 1, 2, and 3, including supportive medical exercise for rehabilitative purposes.

Massage
Massage is a useful adjunct to NMT either as a preparatory intervention to warm-up tissues, to break up stuck or adhered tissues, to increase blood supply, lower sympathetic tone, or to influence fascia. It can be used in the intermediate stage to complement NMT interventions or to finish a treatment.

Massage can be dangerous if used in the wrong or inappropriate situation such as with certain cancer conditions, stroke or osteoporosis to name a few. Some massage techniques such as friction are used to break down fibrotic or scarred tissues and can cause local inflammation. This approach requires much skill and knowledge and should not inflict undue pain on the patient. The notion of sticking an elbow deep into a patient's muscle and frictioning the tissues is enough to make anyone cringe. This is a dangerous and uninformed way to treat tissues. It will in most cases lead to inappropriate tissue damage, irritation, bruising, and increased stress for the patient.

Physical therapists should, when appropriate, make use of t-bars to apply ischemic pressure and/or mild friction rather than developing repetitive strain injury to their own thumbs and fingers. T-bars are relatively inexpensive and can be purchased from the internet. Massage includes variations on the following techniques.

Effleurage
These are generally warming techniques with a broad surface such as the palm of the hands. Techniques can be fast, slow, long, or short, depending on the desired physiological effect. Faster and shorter are stimulating while slower and longer are more relaxing. Other variations include faltering, compressive, or combined. Friction is created between the therapist's hands and the patient's skin. The less oil or cream that is used, the greater the frictioning effect.

Petrissage
These include a multitude of variations including gently lifting muscles up and away from the bones, rolling, and squeezing muscles. Petrissage generally involves kneading and compression motions – rolling, squeezing, or pressing the muscles to enhance deeper circulation. Petrissage helps to stimulate circulation and assists clearing out of energy by-products from muscle and nerve tissue.

Tapotement
This consists of briskly applied percussive movements, using the hands alternately to strike or tap the muscles, to provide an invigorating effect. There are numerous variations on this stroke, which include using the edge of the hand, the tips of the fingers, or with a closed fist. Tapotement attempts to release tension and cramping from muscles in spasm.

Laws of European Neuromuscular Therapy

The neuromuscular therapist provides a physical therapy operating under a system of neurological laws. These laws illustrate both acute and chronic pain patterns and demonstrate how pain is dispersed throughout the body. The nervous system is designed to produce normal muscle tonus at 30 stimuli per second. If the nervous system is suddenly innervating the damaged tissues, due to trauma, at perhaps 75 stimuli per second, it must respond in a more creative homeostatic way to distribute the pain.

The *Law of Unilaterality* states, *"if a mild irritation is applied to one or more sensory nerves, the movement will take place usually on one side only and that side which is irritated."* As an illustration, if a person were involved in a soft tissue insult injuring their left hip and they do not receive treatment, the hip would be painful within a relatively short period of time. Assuming that they continue without treatment and take a pain killer and perhaps a hot shower to ease the pain, not only would the initial injury site still be in pain the following day, but so would the equal and opposite side.

This illustrates the second law, the *Law of Symmetry*; *"if the stimulation is sufficiently increased, the motor reaction is manifested not only to the irritated side but also in similar muscles on the opposite side of the body."* From a practical perspective if a therapist can treat the unaffected side, it is possible that the injured, painful area can be addressed to some degree without initial direct application of NMT.

Without correct treatment of this injury, the pain would now have intensified at the original injury site with a lesser pain present on the contralateral hip. This describes the third law, the *Law of Intensity*, *"reflex movements are usually more intense on the side of irritation and at times the movements of the opposite side equal them in intensity but they are usually less pronounced."*

The fourth law is the *Law of Radiation*, *"if the excitation continues to increase it is propagated upwards and reactions take place through centrifugal nerves coming from the cord segments higher up."* This means the pain will radiate upward from the site of the original injury toward the brain and then, failing alleviation, will radiate outward, creating a general contraction of all the muscles in the body. If left untreated, the patient would at some future date find it difficult to move without pain or be unable to move without intense headache pain, accompanied by a general contraction of all the muscles from their head to toe. The nervous and musculo-skeletal systems would now be adversely affected including all of the other systems in the body, such as the respiratory, cardiovascular, lymphatic, digestive, and endocrine systems.

This illustrates the fifth law, the *Law of Generalization*. This law states, *"if the irritation becomes very intense, it is propagated in the medulla oblongata, which becomes the focus from which the stimuli radiate to all parts of the cord causing a general contraction of all the muscles of the body."* Acute injury (i.e. compression), chronic injury (i.e. repetitive micro trauma), muscle imbalances, joint dysfunctions, and poor posture provide the foundation for negative changes in posture and compromise the integrity of the neural tissues. The neurogenic reflex mechanism is initiated by tissue trauma, as is the cumulative injury cycle. Such changes result in morphological disturbances at the micro level resulting in chemical irritation due to intraneural oedema, tissue hypoxia, microvascular starvation, and the formation of trigger points. Other laws include:

Law of Facilitation
When a neuron takes its course through a specific group of neurons to the exclusion of others it will tend to repeat the same course on future occasions and each time it travels this pathway the resistance decreases. Facilitation occurs when a pool of neurons, (pre-motor neurons, motor neurons or in spinal regions pre-ganglionic sympathetic neurons) are in a state of partial or sub-threshold excitation. This results in a lesser degree of afferent stimulation being required to trigger the discharge of impulses.

Arndt-Schultz's Law
Weak stimuli excite physiologic activity, moderately strong ones favour it and strong ones retard it. Very strong ones arrest it.

Davis' Law

Ligaments or any soft tissue when placed under even a moderate degree of tension will elongate by the addition of new material, if that tension is unremitting. On the contrary, when ligaments or other soft tissues remain uninterruptedly in a loose or lax state, they will gradually shorten, as the effete (by-product) material is removed, until they come to maintain the same relationship to the bony structures with which they are united, that they did before their stretching.

Head's Law

A painful stimulus applied to a body part of low sensitivity (such as an organ) when in close central connection (i.e. the same segmental supply) with an area of higher sensitivity (such as a part of the soma) pain will be felt at the point of higher intensity rather than where the stimulus was applied.

Hilton's Law

A nerve trunk that supplies a joint also supplies the muscles of the joint and the skin over the insertions of those muscles. Each nerve root also serves blood vessels, organs, and glands. Therefore, excitation along a nerve pathway to any of these tissues can spill over to facilitate the other tissues also served by that nerve, creating dysfunction or pain in those secondary tissues as well. For example, excitation to a diseased gallbladder could excite the muscles overlying the area that is innervated by the same nerve that serves that organ.

Hooke's Law

The stress used to stretch or compress a body is proportional to the strain, as long as the elastic limits of the body have not been exceeded.

Sherrington's Law

Every posterior spinal nerve root supplies a specific region of the skin (a *dermatome*) which is invaded above and below by fibres from the adjacent spinal segments.

Wolff's Law

Every change in the form and function of a bone, or in its function alone, is followed by certain definite changes in its internal architecture and secondary alterations in its external conformation; these changes usually represent responses to alterations in weight-bearing stresses.

Neuromuscular Technique

When the term neuromuscular technique (NMTq) is used it should be understood to refer to the technique of assessment and treatment of local musculo-skeletal dysfunction, mainly involving myofascial trigger points, tender points, areas of congestion, scar tissue, fibrosis, oedema, hypersensitivity and numbness utilizing finger and/or thumb techniques.

NMT techniques start in the assessment mode (in the chronic stage) but can, at any stage, move to a treatment mode as the therapist sees fit. NMT is used to identify altered states in the tissues beneath the thumb, or fingers, of the therapist. Digital pressure (ischemic pressure) and strokes are used to locate, identify, and treat focal points. Engaging the tissues by meeting and matching the *return tension* the therapist combs the tissues observing any differences in texture, sensitivity, contour, and pain points whilst encouraging feedback from the patient. In particular a scale should be established (0–10) regarding the level of pain or discomfort or change in sensation experienced by the patient. The therapist should work at a level that causes mild discomfort (5–8) whilst avoiding major pain (9–10 plus).

It is important to avoid rushing when using NMTq. The tissues will begin to melt beneath the therapist's fingers allowing deeper tissues to be palpated and investigated. NMTq is excellent for identifying trigger points as they are located in the muscle fibres. When using the NMT thumb technique, the fingers act as a fulcrum or axis around which the thumb moves.

Search the tissues over a 'four inch' surface area at a time (approx 1.5 seconds every 4 inches) then move the fingers to the next position in whatever direction the therapist wishes to direct the thumb. Forces running through the thumb should run down the long axis of the arm. These forces are generated in the lower limbs and translated through the core to the arm.

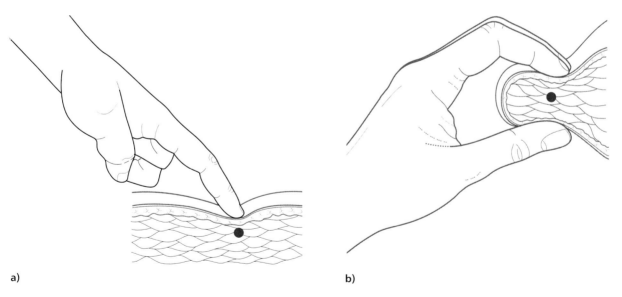

a)   b)

Figure 4.9: a) flat finger palpation, b) pincer palpation.

Muscle Energy Techniques

Muscle energy techniques (MET) are gentle resistive applications where the patient is requested to provide a gentle contraction of specific muscles, from a precisely controlled position in a specific direction, against a mild (25–30%) counterforce for a specific period of time (usually ten seconds). Types of contractions include:

Isometric Contraction
The distance between the origin and insertion remain the same. No movement occurs, the muscle fibres shorten but only initially.

Isotonic Concentric
The length of the muscle shortens. The patient gently overcomes the resistance offered by the therapist.

Isotonic Eccentric
This is also called an *isolytic contraction*, whereby the length of the muscle increases. The patient allows the therapist to overcome their resistance through a specific range of movement. This variation is the most intense and can lead to slight structural damage (if performed correctly) as adhesions are broken down. As already stated some soreness may be expected post-treatment.

MET requires the patient to have the capacity to offer a gentle force against a specific resistance of low intensity provided by the therapist. Having established the first barrier (the first sign of resistance to movement), within a specific range of movement in a specific plane, a number of variations will be used depending on the situation being acute or chronic. In an acute situation, a low intensity contraction is requested from the position where the first sense of restriction is perceived (targeting type 1 fibres).

In the chronic stage this barrier would be avoided and the therapist should back off a small amount to provide the patient with a mechanical advantage. MET is slightly different when a joint is the target. When treating a joint (or in the acute stage) no stretch is employed following a mild contraction.

Most muscle energy procedures use *post-isometric relaxation* (PIR). After an isometric contraction, there is a refractory period during which passive lengthening of the target muscle may be achieved without strong resistance from the target muscle/s due to lowered muscle spindle activity.

Another popular variation on the theme is *reciprocal inhibition*. This takes advantage of the fact that when a target muscle's antagonist is contracted, the target muscle is inhibited and therefore reduces contractile forces. One example of this is a contraction of the quadriceps muscles to inhibit the hamstring muscles.

Indications
- Mobilize restricted joints.

- Return normal length to shortened muscles and fascia.

- Return neuromuscular efficiency to an asymmetrically weak, or inhibited, muscle or to decrease hypertonicity.

- Improve circulation, respiration, and neuromuscular relationships.

- Provide therapeutic input to rectify a more distal pain in the kinetic chain.

Contraindications

MET is not advised if pathology is suspected, for example, a fracture or other serious bone health pathology. The neuromuscular therapist will refer for accurate diagnosis to be established. Once a diagnosis has been confirmed, the correct level or intensity of application can be specifically tailored to suit the particular situation (e.g. arthritis, osteoporosis, etc.).

Following a mild contraction, it is advisable to allow a rest period of about five seconds so that the patient's muscles can reduce in tone and allow for the dissipation of any contractile residue before lengthening. In acute settings the physical therapist should avoid stretching or lengthening the muscle after the contraction phase.

Pulsed MET

This method requires a series of rapid, yet gentle, pulsating contractions against a resistance provided by the therapist. A contraction rate of one every second is usually sufficient. The therapist can work at one specific angle to the joint or move slowly through a range by gently overcoming the patient and slowly moving the limb or body part through a new range of motion. It may be useful to provide some support to the limb to ensure the patient does not overexert. Some body parts are better suited than others regarding this technique. Patients can be instructed to perform this technique at home if appropriate. Stretching of the tissues following the contractile effort is optional. Patients should be encouraged to avoid holding their breath. Correct positioning of the targeted limb will ensure a mechanical advantage and will allow the patient to provide a contraction without additional stress to the tissue or related joint/s.

Upper Crossed Syndrome: A New View

In upper crossed (and indeed the same will apply in lower crossed) syndrome, both the short and lengthened muscles will be weaker than their potential. In other books the muscle relationship in upper crossed syndrome describes one muscle being tight and short, while opposing muscles are weak. It is important to realize that both the short and long muscles will be weak. One muscle will be short, spastic or contractured, and weak while the opposing muscle will be inhibited, lengthened, tight and weak.

Short and Weak

Pectoralis major and minor, upper trapezius, levator scapulae, and sternocleidomastoideus.

Inhibited and Weak

Lower and middle trapezius, deep neck flexors, serratus anterior, and rhomboids.

The following occurs in kinetic chain terms when the upper crossed pattern is noted. Occiput with C1 (atlas) and C2 (axis) hyperextend with the head translating anteriorly. The lower cervical vertebrae down to the fourth thoracic vertebrae are now stressed. Rotation and abduction of the scapula occur as the upper trapezius and levator scapulae become shortened and hypertonic (contracted, contractured, or spastic). As a result of this, the scapula loses stability, which places excess demands on the humerus now involving the levator scapulae, upper trapezius, and supraspinatus to maintain functional efficiency. This will predispose the person to increased risks of rotator cuff injury, shoulder instability, biceps tendonitis, thoracic outlet/inlet syndrome, and headaches.

Further Kinetic Chain Implications

With the neck in hyperextension and the scapula rotated and abducted this rounds out the shoulders and closes down the anterior chest wall reducing the possibility of a full functional breath, and compresses the viscera and abdominal contents. Erector spinae will be inhibited and the deep cervical muscles will be shortened including the anterior and middle scalenes. Short scalenes will have an effect of pulling up the first and second ribs while sternocleidomastoideus pulls the clavicle. This pulling up will be opposed by a pulling down by the psoas muscles causing an internal rotation to the femur and the resulting change in the lower chain and links affecting the position of the feet.

In NMT, we will identify the short muscles first using NMT special tests and then offer interventions that will have a muscle spindle deactivation and GTO response (includes slow, deep ischemic work, MET and PR). The inhibited muscle requires stimulation of the muscle spindles. This work may include placing the target muscle under a stretch and then stimulating or firing up the muscle spindles with up-tempo techniques such as hacking or cupping.

Positional Release (PR) and Strain/Counterstrain (SCS)

Movement is life, and sleeping is an activity involving movement. If you were to see a time lapsed recording of a person sleeping, you would see that sleep is far from being inactive or static. On the contrary, we shift and move 'into' and 'out of' various positions. Many of us start our sleep from some version of the foetal position. During the course of the night, we move many times, rotating, turning, twisting, bending, and so on. In my opinion this is mother natures version of *positional release*. This could be seen as a 'resetting' of the neuromuscular programming, or parameters, after an active day.

Ruffini receptors are located in the joint capsules and report aspects of joint position and velocity as well as direction of movements (see figure 3.12). This information is dealt with by higher brain function within the cerebral cortex and therefore has no direct influence at the local segmental level. The golgi tendon organs (GTOs) and muscle spindles previously mentioned, deal with tension and 'moment to moment' changes in length and velocity (respectively) of muscles. GTOs and muscle spindles are connected directly to the spinal cord by gamma and alpha neurons providing influence specifically at the local spinal level. The muscle spindle is of primary concern in positional release and strain/counterstrain.

Neuromuscular feedback systems including the muscle spindle, GTOs and Ruffini receptors are at the core of many somatic spasm and pain disorders. Ruffini receptors (Rr's) are located within the joint capsule. Rr's are responsive to position, velocity, and direction of motion. Sudden changes in the rate of change in length of muscle lead to larger than normal neural discharges, with tissue tearing, resulting in an immediate contractile response ending in a spastic muscle. The parameters concerning homeostasis specific to the resting length of the muscle will now be changed. Any attempt to lengthen the already short muscle will result in acute intense pain.

In effect the muscle now thinks it is already lengthened and any attempt to increase its length will result in considerable neural loading resulting in pain. This tissue damage leads to the release of chemical substances such as prostaglandins, thromboxanes, leukotrienes, phosphate P, neurotoxins, and monohydroxyl fatty acids. These in turn promote the inflammatory response and consequential hyperalgesia, resulting in vasoconstriction. The local environment now floods with leukocytes, complement activators and the release of pain producing neuropeptides including histamines, serotonin and bradykinines.

Positional release methods ensure a relaxation of the local tissues at the site of the insult or injury. Removal of excessive tension leads to an improvement of blood supply at the specific local level while providing the opportunity to re-set the neuromuscular feedback mechanisms by placing them in a neurological sleep. Increased nutrient blood supply and improved interstitial circulation helps to remove the chemical soup of noxious stimulators and mediators of inflammation. The resulting reduction in tissue tension and guarding reflexes contributes to additional decreases in the release of such substances.

PR and SCS techniques are wonderfully simplistic in their delivery and have amazing potential for restoring pain free range of motion. An individual segment of the spinal cord can become inundated with neural activity.

Neural researchers and experts have stated that if the volume or amplitude of impulses from proprioceptors, nociceptors and higher centres channelled to a specific segment exceeds the capacity of the normal routing pathway, the electrochemical discharges may begin to affect collateral pathways. This, in effect, is what is termed spillover.

Spillover

Spillover of neural activity can be exerted ipsilaterally, contralaterally, or vertically. Impulses arising from any tissue feedback into the local segment can reach a threshold, which once surpassed, begins to be misinterpreted by the central nervous system. Afferent impulses intended to register as pain in the gallbladder can be felt as pain in the shoulder. As stated in this text, the simple reflex arc (stretch reflex, see figure 2.6) is the foundation of many pain syndromes that will not resolve without the hands-on intervention of a qualified physical therapist such as a NMT. Spillover from excessive discharge due to irritated muscle spindle activity and other receptors provides the self-perpetuating source of irritation and pain. Positional release and SCS provide a damping effect on the level of neural excitability within a specific segment allowing the possibility of a return to homeostasis.

In my early years, Leon Chaitow taught me the need to understand numerous variations of PR/SCS to meet the various needs of patients in different settings. In PR/SCS, neuromuscular therapists generally use verbal feedback from the patient (if the patient cannot give verbal feedback, other methods can be employed such as visually indicating the level with one, two or more fingers as appropriate) as to the level or intensity of pain and/or tenderness of a pain point, located with the use of finger or thumb neuromuscular technique. This may, or may not be a trigger point. It may simply be a painful point in a muscle or tissue. The therapist uses this verbal feedback to act as a monitor as they guide the body part or limb into a position of reduced pain and/or ease.

Other methods employed by the neuromuscular therapist do not necessarily rely on verbal feedback but rather the therapist must "plug into" the tissues, palpating, seeking, listening, and recognizing a position of ease with their listening hands or fingers becoming an intelligent extension of their brain. Palpatory skill development is the key to accurate assessment of muscular involvement. Palpation pressure must be consistent throughout the treatment. Pressure is useful for assessment of tender or pain points but is not required during the release or after 16 seconds. A pain point is not always required, such as in positional release variations. Positional release involves the positioning of a patient's limb, limbs, muscle, fascia, or a body part into a position whereby inappropriately tense, hypertonic, short, indurated (spastic) or contractured tissue/s are placed in a position of comfort and away from resistance barriers (bind). This provides the potential for a return of normal neurovascular activity. Achieving this therapeutic response requires expert knowledge of anatomy and palpation skills coupled with knowledge of neurophysiology and circulation. One must appreciate the subtle differences of PR/SCS in order to individualize a treatment strategy unique to the patient's circumstances and needs.

This text will not include all of the many variations of PR/SCS such as mobilization with movement, positional release taping and so on (see Chaitow, L., 2006).

When a sudden unaccustomed increase in muscle length occurs, a combination of neurological and circulatory changes can take place. Due to instant proprioceptive reactions, a change to the resting length of the muscles opposite those that were actively contracting at the time of perceived pain might occur. The resulting muscular spasm is known as the *primary afferent muscle spindle response*. The result is contradictory proprioceptive feedback.

The muscle's proprioceptors now reset their parameters recording the new short status of the muscle as being lengthened. Any attempt to lengthen the now spastic muscle results in a protective reflexive contraction and pain. This spasm creates an ischemic environment depriving the fibres of sufficient oxygen supplies, resulting in hypoxia. Over time, this environment can lead to the formation of trigger points. Vasoneuroactive substances including bradykinin, phosphate P, prostaglandins, and others, create neural sensitization (both spinal-segmental-local) by means of a process known as *facilitation*. Coupled with high levels of inorganic phosphates and lactates, the muscles acidic levels raise causing further hypersensitivity to touch. I refer to this as the *production versus removal dilemma*. When production of certain chemicals far exceeds their removal from a specific site, there is a potential for increased sensitivity. The longer this status is allowed to continue the greater the risk of neural overload, entrapment, and *crosstalk*.

Crosstalk involves axons overloading and passing impulses directly to one another. The result can include spasm, vasomotion, pain impulses, reflex mechanisms, and disturbances in sympathetic activity. A local and global NMT rehabilitation approach is called for. The local approach may involve the use of positional release intervention, muscle energy techniques, trigger point therapy or a gentle combination or synergy of all these. In NMT we refer to this as *integrated neuromuscular inhibition technique* (INIT). Tips on performing quality touch include:

- Take time to position yourself for maximum ease and transference of forces from you to the patient

- Keep the most straight on motion ensuring your pelvis and shoulders are in alignment to your direction of force.

- Place your hands or digital placement gently and search slowly. Keep listening with your hands and fingers.

- Avoid poking or shoving the tissue.

- Ask the patient for movement when applying elbow or digital ischemic pressure to provide additional neural involvement (direct technique).

- A softening or viscosity may occur in the tissues you are working on. Avoid rushing at this stage and watch out for autonomic cues such as a deep breath, blinking, sighing, or other.

- Spend time on releasing the tissues around the bony margins as the deep and superficial fascias merge there.

- Keep a close eye on your patient's reactions and breathing. Working slowly will lead to you synchronizing your work with your patient's breath.

- Position your patient using pillows and bolsters to achieve a sense of floating. This will reduce the amount of force needed to access the deep tissues.

- Visualize the anatomical structures beneath the skin you are working on. This requires excellent knowledge of human anatomy.

- Always apply warm hands and fingers. Avoid cold touch.

"Speed is the enemy"

Uniform Guidelines for PR

- Start with the recommended investigation and assessments including special tests.

- Always ask the patient to first show you or demonstrate their present ROM of the target muscles.

- Evaluate for relative shortness and/or onset of pain.

- Investigate the muscle for a point of pain (this may be a trigger point or simply a painful point).

- Apply ischemic pressure – Ask the patient to report when the level of pain is considered at level 8 out of a possible 10.

- Hold the ischemic pressure for a series of 5 seconds (part 1) with release of the pressure for 2 seconds (part 2).

- Continue this 'two part' cycle until the patient feels their pain level is diminishing. This may involve several cycles, so do be patient.

- Apply ischemic pressure and produce a level of pain between 5 and 8 out of a possible 10 (patient feedback).

- Slowly, and with great sensitivity, begin to passively move the target muscle/limb into a shortened or crowded position.

- Move the muscle/limb towards a position of ease avoiding or backing off any feeling of bind or restriction. Combining palpatory excellence (a listening hand) with patient feedback will lead the therapist to positioning the target muscle into a position of greatest ease or reduced pain (this is usually in the order of a 75% reduction).

- Hold this position with continued ischemic pressure for 16 seconds or without ischemic pressure for 90 seconds.

- Passively return the target muscle/limb to the starting position.

- If appropriate, introduce a mild neuromuscular stretch.

Ten General Rules of PR

1. Follow ease of motion.

2. Move away from pain.

3. Approximate origin and insertion of muscle.

4. Move away from bind or barrier.

5. Recreate the original position of injury or insult.

6. Ensure the patient avoids contracting the target tissue.

7. Palpate for softening of tissues (a listening finger).

8. Find dynamic neutral.

9. Return to the starting position slowly (passive).

10. Incorporate MET as appropriate.

Patient Advice

Patients need to be informed that following any treatment including PR/SCS, a period of altered function may occur with physiological adaptations that can lead to post-treatment soreness. This soreness can last from hours to days. An application of cold water from a shower for 3–6 minutes will provide all the intervention needed to reduce any soreness or discomfort.

Guidelines Concerning Use of Tender Points

Anterior tender points require flexion, lateral flexion, and rotation toward the tender point. Posterior tender points require extension, lateral flexion, and rotation away from the tender point. Choose tender points most proximal and medial and those that seem most painful for primary attention. The most medial tender points require less lateral flexion and rotation. Posterior tender points may need side bending away from the side of the palpated pain point.

Variations

Within NMT, we use the terms *ease* and *bind*. Bind is considered to be the first sign of resistance or undue tension. Ease refers to a lack of antagonistic tension, or restriction, within a range of movement. Two separate procedures involve *direct* and *indirect techniques*. Direct refers to going against the restrictive barrier or bind or as such going *into* the tissue restriction. Indirect involves going away from the restrictive barrier or shortening the tissues.

Exaggeration of the Distortion

This variation is typically used in the acute stage of muscle or soft tissue insults, such as a spasm, whereby a limb is forced into a position of flexion (or extension). Attempts to extend the limb or body part may result in severe pain. In this situation a pain point is not required. This variation requires moving the patient into an exaggeration of the distortion, with fine-tuning involving rotation in one direction or another, until the patient reports a significant reduction of pain, usually in the order of 70–75%. If the perceived pain only reduces by 50%, the therapist may provide additional vectors such as distraction, compression, cold therapy, gentle rocking, or oscillations. At this phase, breath holding in the active or passive phase of respiration for a maximum of three seconds, may prove helpful.

The therapist, who should be using gravitational forces or bolstering effectively, holds the target muscle/limb in this exaggerated position. The patient can be instructed on how to take a limb or muscle into a passive position utilizing bolsters, cushions, or pillows as part of home care. The position can be held for an appropriate period of time, in some cases lasting from 90 seconds to several minutes or even longer.

An addition to this variation is to provide *reciprocal inhibition* (RI) to the target tissues. To do this, the therapist offers gentle resistance (in the order of 50% of available strength), to the patient's opposing muscles (i.e. opposing the target muscle), on returning the affected body part to the neutral position. This approach will contract the opposing muscles and provide the best possible chance of the target tissues returning to normal resting length as muscle spindle activity is dulled throughout the ROM.

This variation on muscle inhibition allows a greater muscular effort than the 25%–30% of effort recommended when contracting the target muscle ensuring we target specific type 1 fibres. In this circumstance, we are contracting the muscle opposite to the target muscle. As this is the case we can use a greater effort to encourage a response that is in proportion to the effort. This is another example of a specific adaptation to an imposed demand.

Replication of the Position of Strain

This is a perfect example of the subtle nature of differentiation within PR. Should the patient remember what they were doing at the time they were injured or felt pain, then this variation may offer the therapeutic intervention required.

Imagine your patient was watching his son (or daughter) playing football. His right foot was placed or resting on a large rock at the level of his left knee and his right forearm was resting on the front of his thigh supporting his weight as he leaned on his right leg. His son (or daughter) suddenly scores a goal and in the excitement he throws his arms and body up and back as his foot slips from the rock and travels at speed toward the ground. The result is a spasm in his hip flexors.

This patient will find he can move further into flexion with ease. Any attempt to move into extension will result in severe pain, usually felt across the lower back. By replicating the position he was in at the time the injury occurred (that is forward flexion), and holding that position with perhaps some fine-tuning, this should result in a beneficial therapeutic outcome returning the tissues to normal or near normal neural activity. The therapist must passively assist the patient's right leg to the floor and in this scenario, the patient can actively extend their torso, contracting gluteus maximus and the erector spinae (among others) offering RI to the target muscles.

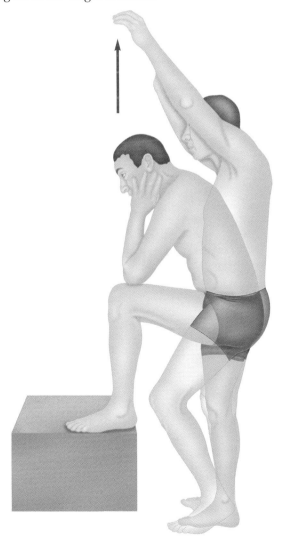

Figure 4.10: Sudden movement causing muscle spasm in psoas and referred pain to the lower back.

Contrary Points Methodology

In this approach, the therapist is encouraged to seek pain points in muscles or tissues opposite those "active" when pain or restriction is noted. Of course this variation will only work provided the patient can remember what they were doing at the time injury occurred. It is worth emphasizing that the pain point is not located in muscles opposite those where pain is noted. So for example, in the case of the biceps brachii, pain would be noted in the elbow, and tender points for treatment would be sought in the triceps brachii (the muscle opposite the one contracting).

In one simplified example, I had a (right handed) patient who presented with a pain in his left shoulder and neck, significantly reduced range of motion and change of sensation down his arm into his third, fourth, and little finger. He also complained of pain in his deltoid. When asked during the initial stage of assessment if he could pinpoint a time and place when his pain problems began, he specified four and a half years previously.

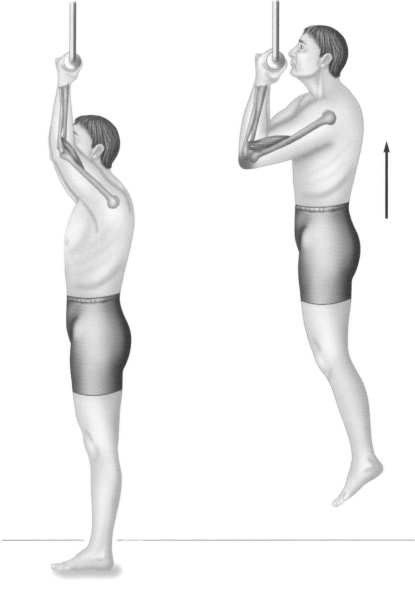

Figure 4.11: Contrary points methodology. In this example, pain is experienced in the elbow as the biceps brachii contract. Tender points for treatment would be sought in the triceps brachii (the muscle opposite the one contracting).

This important input from the patient was the foundation to restoring homeostasis to his muscles. The patient described how he was throwing a tennis ball upwards in a serving action (with his left arm) when still holding the tennis ball (this was vital information). He felt immediate sharp pain in his neck. He lowered his arm, waited a moment or so, and continued on to repeat the motion and this time complete the serve. His problems became more intense over the following days. Over the next four and a half years his pain manifested itself in what seemed a complicated, illogical pattern.

In this case the muscles opposite those that were contracting at the time pain was experienced included latissimus dorsi, teres major, lower trapezius (ipsilateral to the arm holding the ball) and upper trapezius and quadratus lumborum (contralateral to the arm holding the ball). His latissimus dorsi was initially treated and resulted in almost complete restoration of ROM and removal of pain. Subsequent treatments and a medical exercise program helped this patient to return to playing tennis.

Stacking (Functional or Facilitated Technique)

This wonderful variation involves knowledge concerning planes of motion and requires excellent palpatory skills. The therapist engages in a subtle evaluation concerning the quality and range of motion in the target tissues or limb. The focus here is to take the target limb or tissue into what NMT's call *dynamic neutral* (DN). This position is then held and supported by the therapist for an appropriate period of time. This can range from 90 seconds to several minutes. In fact the position of DN could be taped in place and left passively supported for several hours with supportive taping or strapping.

> *"Dynamic neutral is a state in which tissues find themselves when the motion of the structure they serve is free, unrestricted, and within the range of normal physiological limits...Dynamic neutral is not a static condition...it is a continuing state of normal, during living motion, during living activity...it is the state and condition to be restored to a dysfunctional area."*
>
> Chaitow, L. (2006).

An example of this might be a patient with restricted movement in the right glenohumeral joint. The therapist, standing slightly behind and to the right of the patient, places a listening left hand draped across the shoulder joint covering as much surface as possible.

The right hand passively moves the arm in the frontal plane assessing changes in tissue tone and feeling for the first sense of bind in both abduction and adduction until the point of least restriction is found. This point now represents the starting position for the next plane of motion, for instance, flexion and extension in the sagittal plane. Once again, the therapist moving the arm passively and slowly will stop and hold the position of greatest ease or least restriction.

Once more the therapist will move the limb through the next plane offering rotation on the transverse plane. Once the new position of ease has been identified, this can be held for an appropriate period of time (e.g. 90 seconds). Additional vectors such as compression or distraction can be applied. Stacking one plane of motion on top of another provides what we term *dynamic neutral* or the *combined position of ease*. The position of ease is held for an appropriate period of time. This variation can be used in a similar fashion at other joints throughout the body.

Induration Technique

Following a detailed investigation and assessment (if appropriate utilizing NMT thumb or finger techniques and/or skin drag assessment). The therapist can identify tissues of increased *hydrosis*. Hydrosis is a physiological response to increased sympathetic commotion including trigger point activity in the tissues overlying the area of the transverse processes. With the patient lying prone, the therapist stands on the contralateral side to those muscles in which pain has been identified. One hand is used to apply pressure to a pain or trigger point slightly lateral to the lamina groove. The patient scores the pain no more than 8 out of a possible 10.

The opposite hand is used to place its soft thenar eminence lateral to the opposite spinous process most adjacent to the trigger point. Direct pressure towards the pain allows a slackening of the target tissue and pain should begin to reduce. Similar to most PR/SCS methodologies, fine-tuning can be introduced to lower the perceived pain by the recommended minimum of 70–75% or more.

A Note on Ischemic Pressure

Applying pressure to a tissue can significantly reduce blood supply to the tissues directly beneath your finger or thumb. When the pressure is removed, an increase in fresh nutrient rich blood is the desired therapeutic outcome. When you use ischemic pressure to create pain as a feedback mechanism, this author recommends you hold the pressure for no longer than a maximum of 16 seconds. If you choose to hold the tissues in the shortened state for longer than this, remove the ischemic pressure, and if you wish, leave your finger or thumb over the tissue to "listen" and record any changes or reduction in spastic activity.

Ischemic pressure is not always required and in some circumstances is contraindicated. If your patient complains of intensely painful tissues, or perhaps they are too sensitive or fragile, ischemic pressure should be avoided.

Integrated Neuromuscular Inhibition Technique (INIT)

Step one of INIT requires the identification of a trigger point (or simply a pain point) utilizing NM technique and ischemic pressure, if appropriate, within a target muscle.

Step two involves finding dynamic neutral and holding this position of ease for an appropriate period of time.

Step three involves the patient providing an isometric contraction (25–30%) of the target muscle/s at the specific joint angle (*dynamic neutral*) and holding the contraction for no less than 8 seconds and no more than 10. Breath holding is often seen at this stage. Breath holding is of little consequence in young people or patients with no medical history. Be cautious however to encourage your patients with conditions such as high or low blood pressure to avoid holding their breath when contracting muscles or exerting an effort. In step four, the therapist passively moves the target muscle/s into a gentle stretch. Step five, to finish, following a gentle stretch the therapist returns the muscle/s to the resting position.

The tender point can now be re-assessed for comparison and the patient can be instructed to move the limb or body part by gently contracting the targeted muscle/s a few times. Patient feedback is sought with the aim to increase/improve pain-free unrestricted range of motion.

Endless Variations

Once a therapist has gained clinical experience, they can begin to mix and mingle variations as they deem appropriate. Allow yourself to listen to your patient's tissues and they will prompt you as to what they need. This is an intuitive skill, based on excellent knowledge of anatomy, neurophysiology, and palpatory literacy.

Sharkey's Spray and Stretch (Active Cryotherapy Stretching or ACTS)

Caution: Spray and stretch is not always appropriate. Certain muscles or tissues are more suited than others for the application of this powerful technique. Some patients can have adverse reactions to sprays and this should be identified in the screening stage. Care should be taken to ensure that the patient and therapist do not inhale the spray. Spray should not be used without the correct training. Cold spray over the area of the carotid artery and thyroid gland should be avoided.

Slow twitch type 1 muscle fibres, also known as *oxidative* or *aerobic fibres*, contain large numbers of muscle spindles that are sensitive and respond to muscle lengthening. Fast twitch type 2 fibres, also known as *glycolytic* or *anaerobic fibres*, such as gluteus maximus, contain far fewer muscle spindles and therefore have less of a tendency to shorten due to neuromuscular influences manipulated by muscle spindle activity. Having carried out special tests to identify short or spastic muscles, this technique can offer another important option in your ammunition in the war against pain and change in sensation.

Sharkey's spray and stretch technique (ACTS) aims to irritate the spindles, initially, by placing a target muscle into a lengthened position. The patient will feel some discomfort but should not feel inappropriate pain. This stretching will result in the muscle contracting in response to the muscle spindle activity (i.e. a monosynaptic reflex arc). At this stage, the therapist will provide an application of cold spray over the skin in the direction of the lengthened fibres from origin to insertion and further up and down the kinetic chain if deemed appropriate (appropriate care must be taken to avoid damaging the skin or causing an ice burn).

Following the application of the cold spray, the therapist must passively bring the target muscle back to the starting or resting position. A variation could include passively shortening the target muscle beyond its anatomical resting position and holding this position for one or two seconds. Next, the therapist must wipe the skin and dry the area well. This area can now be actively moved, slowly, by the patient to help restore normal neuromuscular parameters.

Sharkey's spray and stretch has shown to be excellent at disassociating adhered tissues but it must be noted that the patient will often feel muscle soreness the following day and possibly for some days later. I first introduced this stretching technique at a fitness instructor conference held in the UK in 1986. At that time it caused quite a stir. After more than twenty years of clinical experience, I recommend it more than ever having witnessed the therapeutic results.

Care must be taken to cover the mouth of the patient (and therapist) to avoid inhaling the spray. The room should be appropriately ventilated and sufficiently large enough to facilitate this procedure. Some individuals have been known to react badly to the topical application of creams, oils and/or sprays. Ask about this during the assessment stage.

It is strongly recommended that all therapists should have appropriate knowledge of emergency first aid and a system in place for effectively dealing with such an event. A wet ice cube can be used as an alternative, moving the wet ice cube up and down the targeted muscle while under stretch. Ice should never be applied directly to skin in the first instance. Avoid static application of the ice in this specific situation. By wetting the ice cube, therefore allowing it to melt a little, the risk of an ice burn is avoided. The therapist should avoid holding the ice cube directly but rather use tissue paper to hold the ice between their fingers, to avoid the risk of damage.

Connective Tissue Release (CTR) (aka known as Soft Tissue Release (STR))

This is a wonderful and versatile technique with many variations on the theme. As discussed previously, *critical fibre distance* (CFD) needs to be maintained to ensure full range of motion and ease of movement without restriction. CTR/STR requires knowledge of a muscle's origin, insertion, tendon type (or aponeurosis), and muscle fibre direction. Muscle fibres can become adhered to each other and muscles can, in turn, adhere to neighbouring muscles, structures, or fascia.

CTR/STR aims to trap a portion of tissue (*connective tissue lock*) and move the remaining tissue below the connective tissue lock, including any fibres contained within the tissue, into a stretch position. The application of the spatula portion (or indeed any other portion) of a thumb, finger (or elbow) into a muscle, locking down the tissue directly beneath the digit (or elbow), ensures a specific point from where the application of ischemic pressure is combined with a lengthening force, either passively (therapist) or actively (patient moves the limb or body part).

Starting superficially and working deeper, the therapist repeats the application of connective tissue lock and lengthening movement providing a unique rhythm, or pace, that meets and matches that of the adhered tissue beneath the listening finger or elbow. This application aims to improve range and quality of motion by breaking up the adhesive relationships of once autonomous fibres or tissues. The very nature of CTR/STR leads to minor tissue damage and inflammation. Patients must be informed that following this treatment, typically within twelve to twenty hours, muscles will be sore. This is temporary and will reduce and subside within a day or so.

CTR/STR is complemented by gently providing effleurage to the target muscles either pre- or post-treatment. The use of oil or cream is optional and the therapist may find they can engage, grip, or lock into the tissue more effectively through a light towel or directly to the skin by reducing the amount of lubricant used.

A wonderful variation on this technique is the application of broad based pressure applied by anterior surfaces of the distal phalanges to encourage a broadening of the muscle fibres during the concentric contraction phase of muscular activity. The simplest example is to describe a patient sitting on the end of a massage table (plinth). The therapist places the anterior aspect of the distal phalanges (one or both hands, preferably both) onto the patient's quadriceps, with their thumbs touching, applying gentle pressure with the knee in flexion. On command, the patient extends the leg at the knee joint whilst the therapist rotates their arms into outward rotation. The muscle fibres will move apart as the muscle contracts.

The added gentle assistance from the therapist is a powerful additional intervention to encourage critical fibre distance. Fingers, thumbs, and elbows can be used in different body regions in targeting more precise, or smaller numbers of fibres.

Contraindications

Any bone pathology, muscle tears, or open skin.

Mechnotherapy (Body Mobilization or Harmonic Technique)

Mechnotherapy involves controlled passive oscillations and gentle vibrations (provided by the therapist) through the connective tissue elements and joints. This provides the opportunity for the patient with high sympathetic tone to "let go". Similar to the way one would gently shake free a bundle of electrical wires that had become wrapped up in each other, with cyclical rhythmic motion. Mechnotherapy offers a gentle unwinding of muscle fibres. The therapist must move the body part, or structure, by starting slowly, building up to a rhythmic motion and resonance that is dictated by, and in tune with, the patient's own tissues.

This technique can be used as a diagnostic tool for identifying areas of excessive tissue tension and restrictions. By placing one hand (e.g. right hand) on the patient's sacrum while they are in the prone position, the therapist can offer a full body rocking, gently allowing the soft tissues to "wobble" on the osseous tissues. Using their free hand, the therapist can place the hand over the moving tissues "listening" and comparing freedom and quality of movement of left to right. The therapist can confirm their findings visually. A slight change in position of a limb such as internal or external rotation or the introduction of a bolster strategically placed or wedged beneath a joint can provide the correct intervention to allow the unrestricted flow of the energy provided by the oscillations.

Use of Oils, Creams, Sprays, and Lotions

To avoid the risk of anaphylactic episodes, the therapist must ensure that their patient has no known adverse reaction to topical applications. In any circumstance, a small sample of the oil or cream to be used (if needed) can be applied to the surface of the skin before a larger amount is applied. A common mistake made by therapists concerns the application of heat creams. One can imagine that depending on the circumstances, for example a pre-event massage scenario, a therapist could apply some heat producing topical cream. Some individuals and athletes look for such applications before a competition.

The problem lies in the fact that one application to one individual is fine but if the therapist is applying the cream to several people they too are absorbing the cream into their body with each application. Steps need to be taken to avoid this.

Note

Always consult an athlete's doctor, trainer, or coach regarding the use of any creams, sprays, or oils. It has been known that some oils, creams or sprays unwittingly contain banned substances. It is often best if the athlete provides you with a cream or oil of his or her own choice.

Review of the Major Skeletal Muscles

5

Muscles of the Face, Head, and Neck

Muscles of the Trunk

Muscles of the Shoulder, Arm, and Hand

Muscles of the Hip and Thigh

Muscles of the Leg and Foot

Red areas highlight the most common sites of referred pain/changes in sensation. For a more detailed description, refer to the text under the heading *trigger point comment*

Referred pain patterns associated with specific trigger point(s)

Derivation of the muscle name

The attachment that remains relatively fixed during muscular contraction

The attachment that moves

Movement or effect caused when the muscle contracts

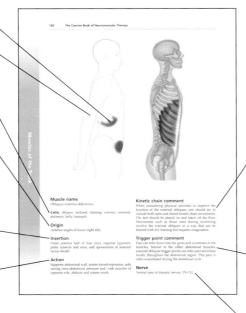

Individual muscles are one link in a chain of muscles responsible for producing any movement

Reported pain referral patterns and sensations specific to each muscle

Nerve(s) that activates the muscle

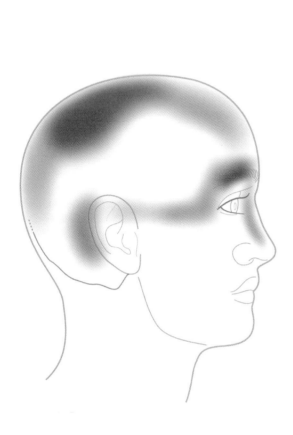

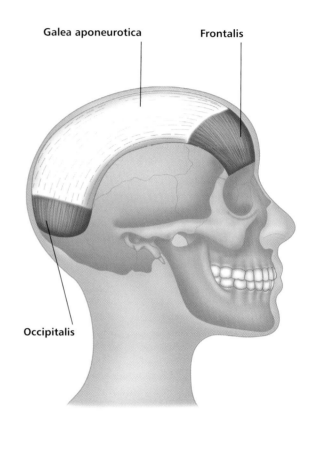

Galea aponeurotica   Frontalis

Occipitalis

Muscle name
Epicranius (occipitofrontalis).

Greek, *epi-*, upon; **Latin**, *cranium*, skull.

Origin
Occipitalis: Lateral two-thirds of superior nuchal line of occipital bone. Mastoid process of temporal bone.
Frontalis: Galea aponeurotica.

Insertion
Occipitalis: Galea aponeurotica.
Frontalis: Fascia and skin above eyes and nose.

Action
Occipitalis: Moves the scalp backward. Assists frontal belly to raise eyebrows and wrinkle forehead.
Frontalis: Moves the scalp forward and wrinkles the skin of the forehead horizontally.

Kinetic chain comment
This is essentially two muscle gastors with a strong fascial connection called the *galea aponeurotica*. Spasm in muscles such as the hamstrings (e.g. biceps femoris) or the plantar fascia can cause tightness through this area ultimately causing tension in the head and neck, or cause headaches. Tension anywhere along the posterior back line kinetic chain can result in shortening of the galea aponeurotica resulting in tension headaches and hyperextended cervical spine. This can result in a posteriorly tilted pelvis to provide a level eye view when walking or running. This is a recipe for trigger point formation.

Trigger point comment
Pain is referred upwards from the frontalis over the forehead on the same side. Occipitalis can refer pain into the eyeball or behind the eye. Pain can travel down behind the ear and into the nose. Sensitivity to sound and light are reported with a resulting increase in experienced pain. This author has had patients who complained of severe pain "inside their head". On investigation, trigger points in the occipitalis reproduced a recognisable pain.

Nerve
Facial V11 nerve.

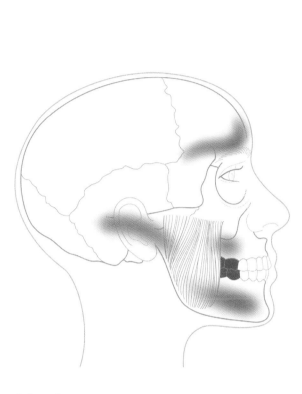

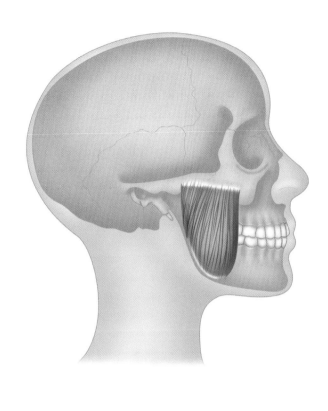

Muscle name
Masseter.

Greek, *maseter*, chewer.

Origin
Zygomatic process of the maxilla and anterior two-thirds of the zygomatic arch (superficial portion). Deep surface of the zygomatic arch (deep portion).

Insertion
Angle of the mandible and outer surface of the ramus (superficial) and coronoid process of the mandible.

Action
Closes jaw. Elevation of the mandible and slight protraction of the jaw.

Kinetic chain comment
Forward head posture places the mandible in a position that puts the masseter under undue stress. Antagonist muscles such as geniohyoid, omohyoid, and digastric can all become spastic due to overtraining of the abdominal muscles using poor technique. This in turn may inhibit masseter with resulting trigger point formation to provide stiffness or tension within the muscle. Learning to train the abdominals with correct technique could restore normal muscle function.

Changes in associated suboccipital muscles lead to changes in homeostasis of the head and face muscles. Change in the positioning of the temporomandibular joint will also affect the position of the cervical spine. Correct alignment of the temporomandibular joint requires treatment of the masseter and pterygoids at the local level with attention to core efficiency at the global level. The ideal solution is the combination of neuromuscular therapy supported with appropriate, graded medical exercise.

Trigger point comment
Masseter is a complex muscle, and pain is referred into the eyebrow, maxilla, mandible (anterior) and to the upper and lower molar teeth. Any person with a toothache will rightly go to a dentist. With no obvious pathology presenting, it is in the patient's best interests to rule out the possibility of referred pain from trigger points being at the root of the pain. Other related sensations include hypersensitivity to pressure and temperature changes (e.g. during flights). Pain can also refer into the temporomandibular joint and inner ear. Remember it is not always about pain. Masseter trigger points are significant contributors to headaches.

Nerve
Trigeminal V nerve (mandibular division).

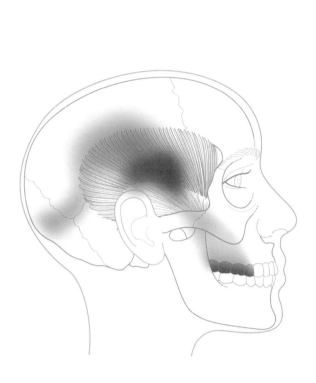

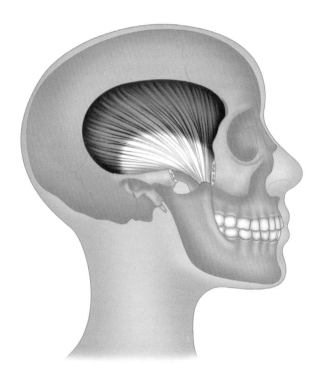

Muscle name
Temporalis.

Latin, pertaining to the lateral side of the head, time.

Origin
Deep surface of the temporal fascia and the entire fossa. The floor of the fossa is made up of the zygomatic, frontal, parietal, sphenoid and temporal bones.

Insertion
Medial/lateral apex and deep surfaces of the coronoid process of the mandible and anterior border of the ramus of the mandible.

Action
Closes jaw (elevates mandible), assists side to side deviations of the mandible and clenching of the teeth. Pulls the ears up to create tension across the scalp.

Kinetic chain comment
Temporalis is a synergistic muscle to masseter. Overdeveloped upper trapezius can be an overlooked contributor to problems associated with this muscle. Short temporalis leads to teeth clenching which can damage the sensitive proprioceptive covering on the teeth. Temporal dysfunction can ensue with loss of balance, vertigo, nausea, hearing difficulties, tinnitus, trigeminal neuralgia, and optical problems. The neck, face, and head muscles are as important to global muscle function as the core (LPH). Habits such as chewing gum can cause repetitive stress and strain. This is an important muscular link in the lateral chain, and spasm in this muscle can play havoc on the positioning of the temporomandibular joint. Short spastic temporalis can reduce the normal ebb and flow of cerebral spinal fluid, inhibiting other muscles. Neuromuscular intervention is called for in this instance.

Trigger point comment
As temporalis is a synergistic muscle to masseter, one can appreciate the chain effect that an inhibited masseter could have on this muscle. Temporalis and masseter may develop trigger points to provide tension to conteract the pulling forces of the excessive tension in the supra- and infrahyoids pulling the jaw down. Forward head posture is again most likely the evident posture. Pain passes upwards and over the forehead on the ipsilateral side. Pain can spillover just above the ear and into the nuchal line of the occiput. This muscle should be considered in all headache patients. Pain in the upper or lower teeth and gums is the most common pain pattern with temporalis. A deep pain has also been reported over the eyebrow and occasionally into the same side and back of the head. Treatment of other muscles based on their pain referral pattern, if associated to this area, must also be treated as part of the myokinetic chain.

Nerve
Anterior and posterior deep temporal nerves from the trigeminal V nerve (mandibular division).

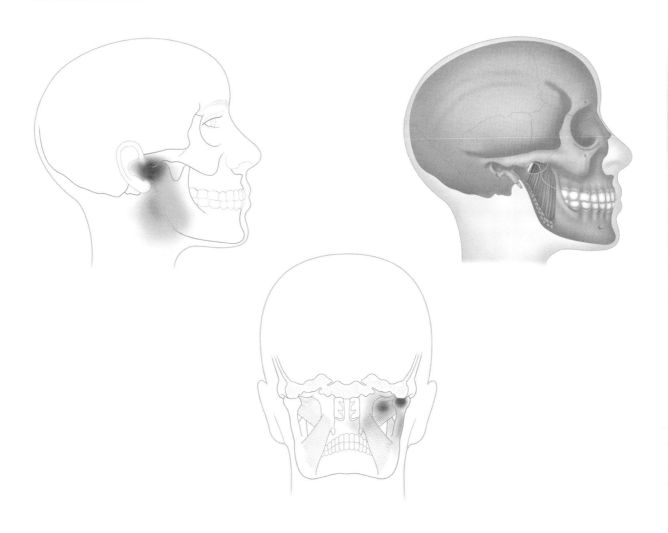

Muscle name
Pterygoid medialis.

Greek, *pterygodes*, like a wing; **Latin**, *medius*, middle.

Origin
The deep head originates on the medial side of the lateral pterygoid plate behind the upper teeth, and the superficial head on the maxillary tuberosity.

Insertion
Both insert onto the medial (fovea) angle of the mandible.

Action
Acts to elevate the mandible, close the jaw, and help the pterygoideus lateralis in moving the jaw from side to side.

Kinetic chain comment
Lower limb length inequalities cause mechanical stress which has been associated with trigger point formation in muscles of the neck, especially sternocleidomastoideus. Sternocleidomastoideus in turn can be the site of mummy or daddy trigger points that form baby or satellite trigger points in the pterygoids. The author does not encourage efforts to strengthen this muscle with resisted protrusion and static stretching. This I believe can offer short-term removal of symptoms but long-term reinforcement of the problems. A focus on removing trigger points is vital but must be followed by a program of physical activity involving neuromuscular full body kinetic chain movement.

Trigger point comment
Pain is referred deep into the temporomandibular joint and maxillary sinus. These trigger points are most often mistaken for arthritis or sinusitis. Pain has also been reported to be a causative factor in tinnitus. Also, pain can be experienced in the tongue and the back of the mouth with difficulty swallowing.

Nerve
Trigeminal V nerve (mandibular division).

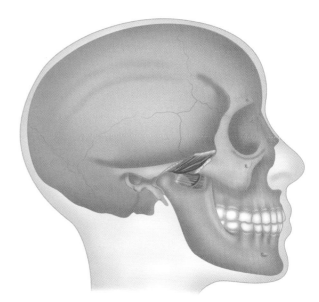

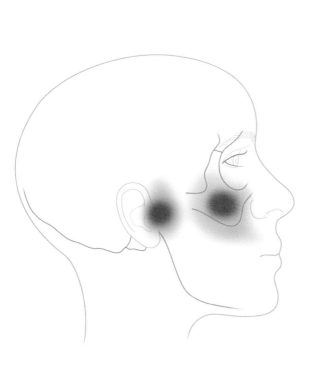

Muscle name
Pterygoid lateralis.

Greek, *pterygodes*, like a wing; **Latin**, *lateral*, to the side.

Origin
Superior head attaches to lateral surface of greater wing of sphenoid, and inferior head of lateral pterygoid plate of sphenoid.

Insertion
Capsule and articular disc of the temporomandibular joint and neck of mandible.

Action
Opens the mouth, protrudes the mandible and provides side to side movement.

Kinetic chain comment
Lower limb length inequalities, including a hemipelvis, cause mechanical stress which has been associated with trigger point formation in muscles of the neck, especially sternocleidomastoideus. Sternocleidomastoideus in turn can be the site of mummy or daddy trigger points that form baby or satellite trigger points in the pterygoids. The author does not encourage efforts to strengthen this muscle with resisted protrusion and static stretching. This I believe can offer short-term removal of symptoms but long-term reinforcement of the problems. A focus on removing trigger points is vital but must be followed by a program of physical activity involving neuromuscular full body kinetic chain movement.

Trigger point comment
Pain is referred deep into the temporomandibular joint and maxillary sinus. These trigger points are most often mistaken for arthritis or sinusitis. Pain has also been reported to be a causative factor in tinnitus. Also, pain can be experienced in the tongue and the back of the mouth with difficulty swallowing.

Nerve
Trigeminal V nerve (mandibular division).

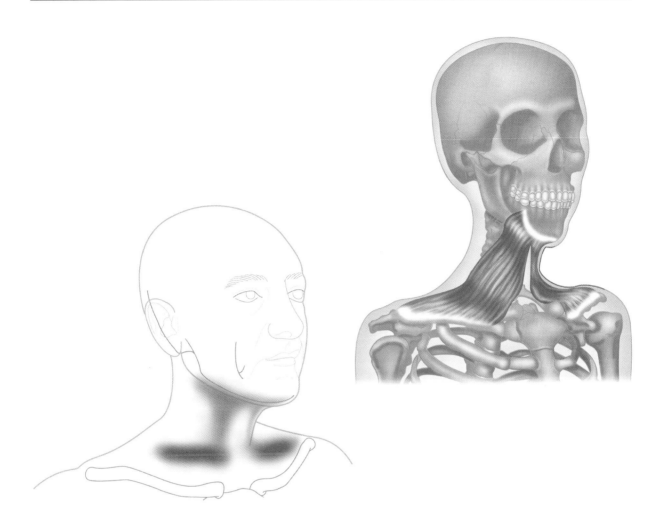

Muscle name
Platysma.

Greek, *platy*, broad, flat.

Origin
Skin and superficial fascia of the neck and upper quarter of the chest and sometimes out to the shoulder.

Insertion
Subcutaneous fascia of the chin and jaw, including the associated muscles.

Action
Assists in opening the mouth and produces an expression of effort or horror. Pulls the lower lip from corner of the mouth down and out to the side.

Kinetic chain comment
This is a muscle of the integumentary system and is used by horses to shake off irritating insects. Hypertension in this muscle pulls the mouth downward and the thoracic skin forward. It is recommended that tissues overlying the thyroid gland might have an influence on glandular function, and so should be examined when glandular dysfunctions are noted. Referral is recommended. This muscle is often punished when exerting fatigue sets in, due to neuromuscular inefficiency or lack of fitness leading to strain being placed on platysma. Short tight masseter can inhibit platysma leading to teeth grinding, especially during sleep.

Trigger point comment
Hot prickling pain in the upper chest and under the jaw bone can be the result of trigger points in this integumentary muscle. Fibres of platysma blend into associated muscles of the face and upper chest wall such as orbicularis oris (mouth), subclavius, and the pectorals. Trigger points can develop, provoking anterior throat stiffness and increased blinking of the eyelids.

Nerve
Facial nerve V11 (cervical branch).

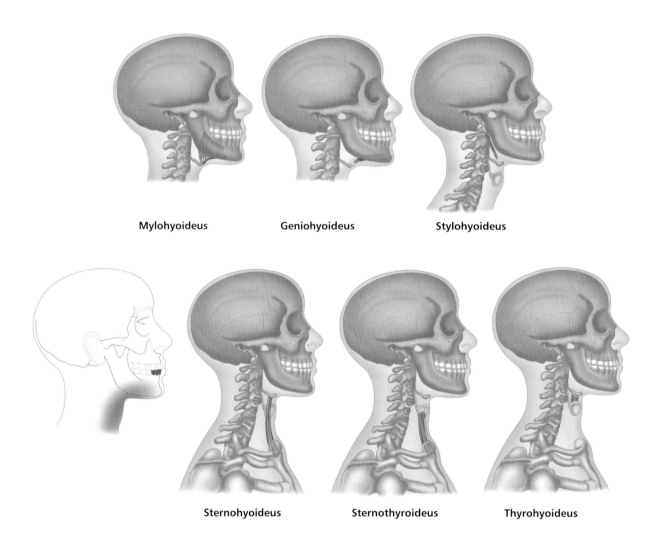

Mylohyoideus   Geniohyoideus   Stylohyoideus

Sternohyoideus   Sternothyroideus   Thyrohyoideus

Muscle name
Hyoids.

Greek, *hyoeides*, shaped like the Greek letter upsilon (v).

Origin
The many muscles of the hyoid group have attachments to the mandible, temporal, manubrium, clavicle, the costal cartilage of the first rib, and the thyroid cartilage.

Insertion
Hyoid bone.

Action
All of these muscles have an effect on the positioning of the hyoid bone. In particular they offer stiffness to stabilize the hyoid when other muscles are carrying out some function.

Kinetic chain comment
The mylohyoideus, sternohyoideus, omohyoideus, geniohyoideus, sternothyrohyoideus, thyrohyoideus, stylohyoideus, and digastric (indirect attachment) muscles all contract to hold the hyoid in place when performing supine sit-ups. They can only do this if the tongue, which also attaches to the hyoid with no origin, is held in its physiological resting position in the roof of the mouth.

Trigger point comment
Trigger points can form in these muscles, referring pain into the lower front teeth and throughout the cervical spine, mostly anterior neck pain. This author suggests that trigger points can develop in the hyoids due to inhibited transversus abdominis and obliquus internus abdominis coupled with spastic sternocleidomastoideus and suboccipital muscles due to faulty training.

Nerve
Ansa cervicalis nerve, C1–C3.

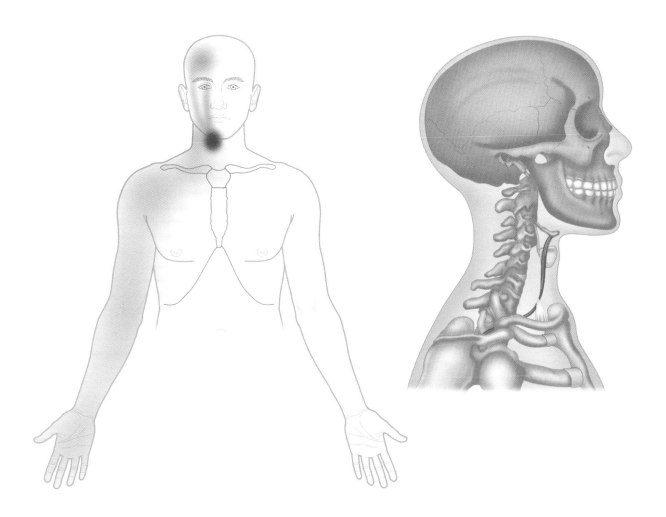

Muscle name
Omohyoideus.

Greek, *omos*, shoulder; *hyoeides*, shaped like the Greek letter upsilon (v).

Origin
Posterior gastor: Mastoid notch on the mastoid process of the temporal bone.
Anterior gastor: Inferior border of the mandible.

Insertion
By means of a common tendon to the hyoid bone.

Action
Depresses the hyoid bone.

Kinetic chain comment
This muscle can literally pick up the lungs as its superior transverse ligament has a fascial connection to the apex of the lungs. The hyoids are important muscles in forced inspiration. If they cannot provide the necessary forces, it is easy to assume an individual would have difficulty improving their aerobic fitness or have difficulty in breathing when under stress or increased intensity due to physical activity. Eccentrically decelerates tilting the head to the contralateral side and depression of the scapula.

Trigger point comment
Patients often complain of sore throats and difficulty in swallowing. My experience has been this muscle can send pain into the shoulder and up into the head on the same side. Tenderness on the hyoid bone itself is noted. Pain in the shoulder, neck, arm, and hand, and in the scapular, supraclavicular, mandibular, and temporal regions may be caused by the omohyoideus. This may be primary, caused by vomiting or by other intense use of the muscle. Caution, trigger points may be secondary, occurring as a result of rheumatoid myositis, ankylosing spondylitis, nonankylosing rheumatoid spondylitis, gouty myositis, or other disorders, which should be ruled out in the first instance.

Nerve
Ansa cervicalis nerve, C2, 3.

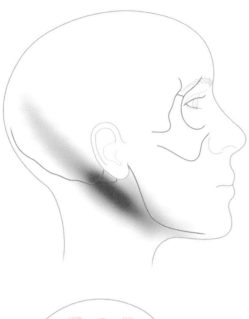

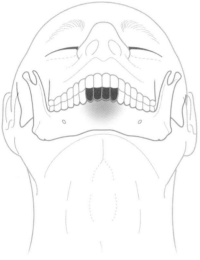

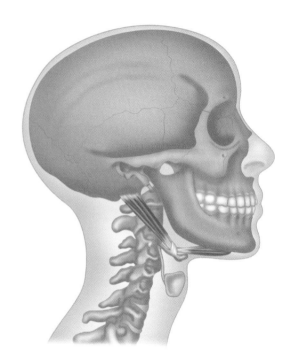

Muscle name
Digastricus.

Latin, having two bellies.

Origin
Anterior belly: Digastric fossa on inner side of lower border of mandible, close to symphysis.
Posterior belly: Mastoid notch of temporal bone.

Insertion
Body of the hyoid bone by means of a fascial sling over its intermediate tendon.

Action
Raises the hyoid bone. Depresses and retracts mandible.

Kinetic chain comment
This muscle must be allowed to create appropriate tension during movements such as crunches or sit-ups. When the tongue is not placed in its physiological resting position, digastricus cannot create this tension resulting in sternocleidomastoideus having to stiffen and shorten. This results in forward head posture and leading to trigger points down the kinetic chain.

Trigger point comment
Pain is experienced in the front teeth, anterior jaw bone, and into the upper part of sternocleidomastoideus (occasionally onto the base of the occiput) and into the throat under the chin. Digastric trigger points have been reported to be responsible for satellite trigger points in the occipitofrontalis and referring pain into the ear.

Nerve
Anterior belly: Mylohyoid nerve, from trigeminal V nerve (mandibular division).
Posterior belly: Facial (VII) nerve.

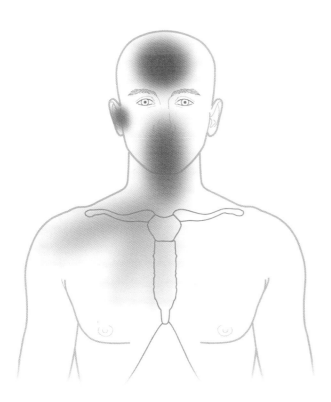

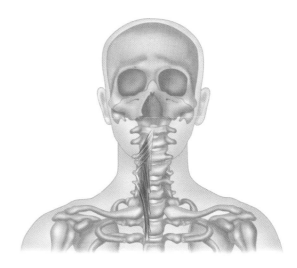

Muscle name
Longus colli.

Latin, *longus*, long; *colli*, of the neck.

Origin
The longus colli has three specific parts (superior oblique, inferior oblique, vertical) lying on the anterior lateral aspect of both the upper cervical and thoracic vertebrae. Ranging from the transverse processes of the third, fourth, and fifth cervical vertebrae with attachments to the anterior aspects of the first two cervical vertebrae and including the anterior surface of the first three thoracic vertebrae.

Insertion
The anterior tubercle of the atlas and anterior tubercles of the transverse processes, C5, 6.

Action
Bilaterally flexes the cervical spine while unilateral contraction assists in rotation to the opposite side and lateral neck flexion.

Kinetic chain comment
Longus colli can become short and tight due to inappropriate neck movements resulting in short scalenes, short tight psoas in turn affecting the action of the diaphragm resulting in trigger point formations causing neck, upper back, and lower back pain. Poor technique during repetitive exercise can result in kinetic chain problems linking the longus colli in the neck to the peroneals on the lateral aspect of the lower limb, possibly resulting in fallen arches. Decelerates extension of the neck bilaterally and unilaterally decelerates ipsilateral rotation and lateral neck extension.

Trigger point comment
Common problem with swallowing, pain in the anterior neck, mouth, ear, and head, and a feeling of a lump in the throat. Patients may complain of a sore throat. This author has experienced trigger points that refer pain across the upper chest on the affected side to the ipsilateral deltoid and a feeling of tightness across the chest. Also, patients report pain across the anterior clavicle and into the tongue. Short spastic psoas can have a significant effect on the development of trigger points in longus colli and associated muscles of the neck. Local pain reported as a deep, thin, and acute sensation at the vertebral level raising up to the eye on the ipsilateral side. Longus colli can be the true source of sternocleidomastoideus pain and is worth considering for treatment in sternocleidomastoideus pain issues.

Nerve
Ventral rami of cervical nerves, C2–C7.

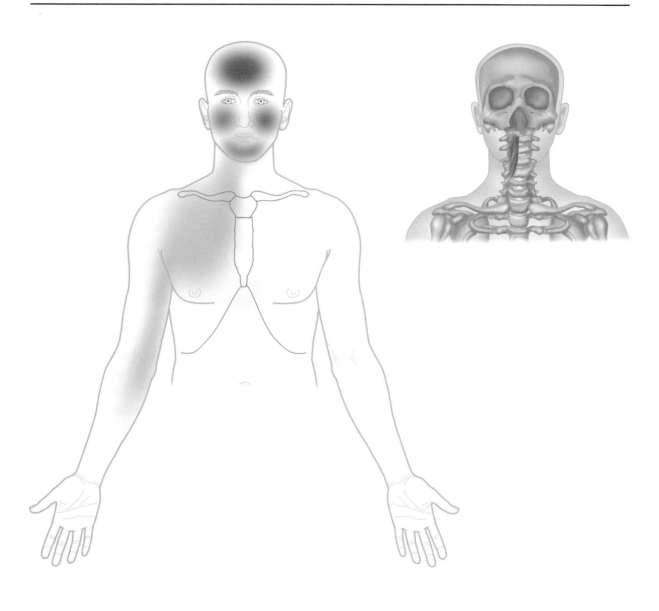

Muscle name
Longus capitis.

Latin, *longus*, long; *capitis*, of the head.

Origin
Anterior tubercles of the transverse processes of the third, fourth, fifth, and sixth cervical vertebrae.

Insertion
Inferior surface of basilar portion of the occiput.

Action
Flexes the neck and superior portion of the cervical spine.

Kinetic chain comment
Longus capitis decelerates neck extension. It may be worth treating short psoas muscles as part of treating longus capitis, as trigger points can be as a response to spasm in the lower chain muscles.

Trigger point comment
Longus capitis can contribute to general pain in the head, face, teeth, and jaw while referring pain down the arm and chest wall. Patients experience pain in the front of the throat, and complain of difficulty swallowing. A feeling of a lump in the throat and sinus type pain is reported.

Nerve
Ventral rami of cervical nerves, C1–C4.

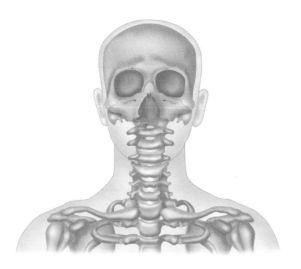

Rectus capitis anterior

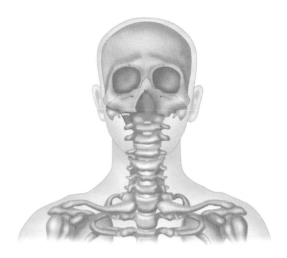

Rectus capitis lateralis

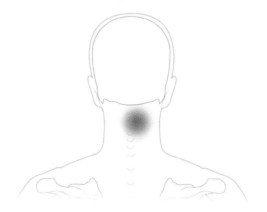

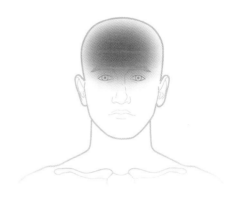

Muscle name
Rectus capitis (anterior, lateralis).

Latin, *rectum*, straight; *capitis*, of the head; *anterior*, before; *lateral*, to the side.

Origin
Anterior: Anterior surface of the lateral mass of the atlas.
Lateralis: Transverse process of the atlas.

Insertion
Anterior: Basilar portion.
Lateralis: Jugular process.

Action
Anterior: Flexes the head.
Lateralis: Lateral flexion to the same side.

Kinetic chain comment
Decelerates the head during extension and contralateral flexion. Spasm or shortness in this muscle can set up the foundation for retarded proprioceptive facilitation and a tendency to collide with objects, get timing wrong, and reduce accuracy. Attention should be paid to sternocleidomastoideus and head position in conjunction with a focus on the posterior myofascial chain. Remember from a kinetic chain viewpoint the true source of rectus capitis dysfunction could be held as far away as the plantar fascia.

Trigger point comment
Trigger points in this muscle have been reported to cause brain pain (or intensify the pain of true migraines). This can feel like severe migraine type pain everywhere inside the head. Patients may say they cannot pinpoint the pain but feel it widespread throughout the cranium. Like other posterior neck muscles, these trigger points can contribute to painful tension-like or cervicogenic headaches. Eyes become sensitive to bright light and patients experience difficulty in concentrating. Pain in the posterior neck and lower intolerance to touch. Change in sensations can include numbness, tingling, and burning in the scalp. Trigger points can reduce or retard blood flow and impede nerve tissue.

Nerve
Loop between ventral rami of cervical nerves, C1, 2.

Muscles of the Face, Head, and Neck

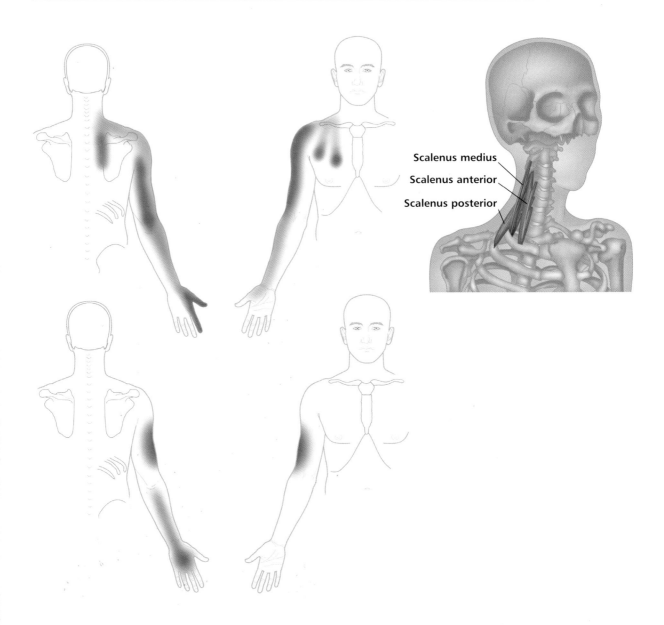

Scalenus medius
Scalenus anterior
Scalenus posterior

Muscle name
Scalenes.

Greek, *skalenos*, uneven.

Origin
Transverse processes of all cervical vertebrae.

Insertion
First rib and/or suprapleural membrane. The posterior portion may attach to the first two ribs.

Action
Elevates the ribs for respiration if ribs are fixed. Rotates to the side opposite of the muscle contracting. Laterally flexes to the contracted side. Bilaterally flexes the neck.

Kinetic chain comment
Trigger points causing short psoas muscles can lead to adaptations in the scalenes muscles resulting in a short contracted state pulling up the rib cage and affecting respiratory efficiency.

Trigger point comment
Pain and numbness can be experienced in the anterior chest, upper back, lateral-anterior shoulder down the arm radiating into the thumb and fourth finger. These are a complex group of muscles with varying muscle fibre length and therefore with potential for many trigger points. Excellent palpatory skills will be required to successfully locate such trigger points.

Nerve
Ventral rami of cervical nerves, C3–C8.

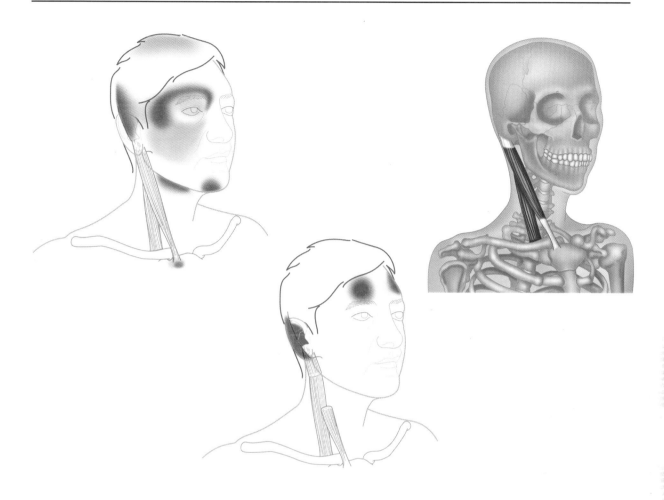

Muscle name

Sternocleidomastoideus (SCM).

Greek, *sternon*, sternum; *kleidos*, key, clavicle; *mastoid*, breast-shaped, mastoid process.

Origin

Manubrium of the sternum and medial portion of the clavicle (two heads).

Insertion

Mastoid process of the temporal bone.

Action

Rotates to side opposite that contracting and laterally flexes to the contracted side. Bilaterally flexes the cervical spine (neck).

Kinetic chain comment

Generally speaking, the muscle most people feel hurting or tense when performing sit-ups. When short, changes the position of the head on the neck resulting in forward head posture (FHP). FHP sets up the foundation for kinetic chain pain and postural changes leading to compensation, change of gait, and decompensation. Rounded shoulders often have their roots in short sternocleidomastoideus.

Trigger point comment

Sternocleidomastoideus are a complex muscle group, not just creating referred pain, but includes problems with balance, visual difficulties, and systemic symptoms. Due to their anatomical position, SCM trigger points can be mistaken for swollen glands. Referred pain can be felt as a headache across the front of the brow, deep eye pain (involving decreased or blurred vision), pain on swallowing, pain behind the ear (including a degree of deafness) and in the top (crown) of the head. I have had patients with SCM trigger points who had pain similar to trigeminal neuralgia. Such pain can be diagnosed as sinusitis. Rare pain referral can also include toothache in the back molars and pain on the opposite side of the forehead. Pain in the manubrium of the sternum has also been reported. Pain is referred to the temples, tongue, throat, and to the side of the neck in some patients.

Nerve

Accessory XI nerve; with sensory supply for proprioception from cervical nerves, C2, 3.

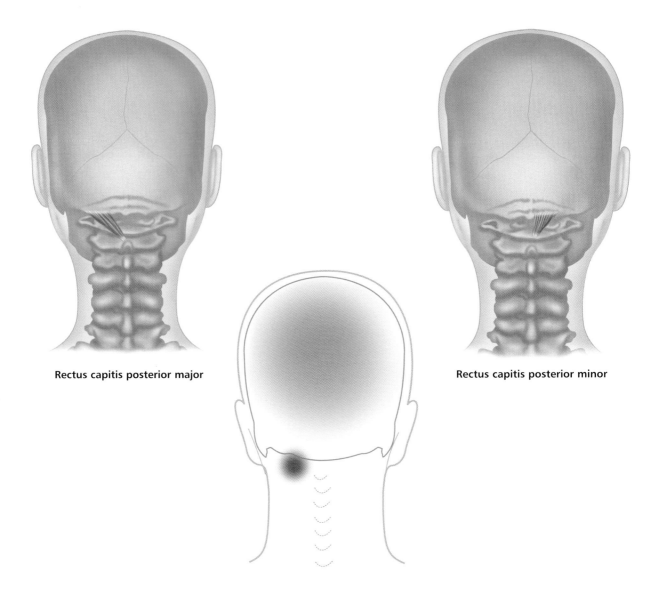

Rectus capitis posterior major

Rectus capitis posterior minor

Muscle name
Rectus capitis posterior (major, minor).

Latin, *rectum*, straight; *capitis*, of the head; *posterior*, behind; *major*, large; *minor*, small.

Origin
Posterior process of atlas (C1).

Insertion
Medial half of inferior nuchal line.

Action
Extends and rotates atlanto-occipital joint.

Kinetic chain comment
These muscles are vital for reporting the position of the body in time and space. Rich with muscle spindles, their role is as much about sending information to the brain regarding head position, as it is about creating movement. With fascial attachments to the spinal cord and brain via the dura mater, these muscles are vital in spinal health and the healthy flow of cerebrospinal fluid.

Trigger point comment
Mimicking migraine pain, these muscles often create what many patients refer to as brain pain. A pain felt deep in the head but the patient cannot put their finger on where the pain is exactly. Migraine pain has often been attributed to this muscle.

Nerve
Suboccipital nerve (dorsal ramus of first cervical nerve, C1).

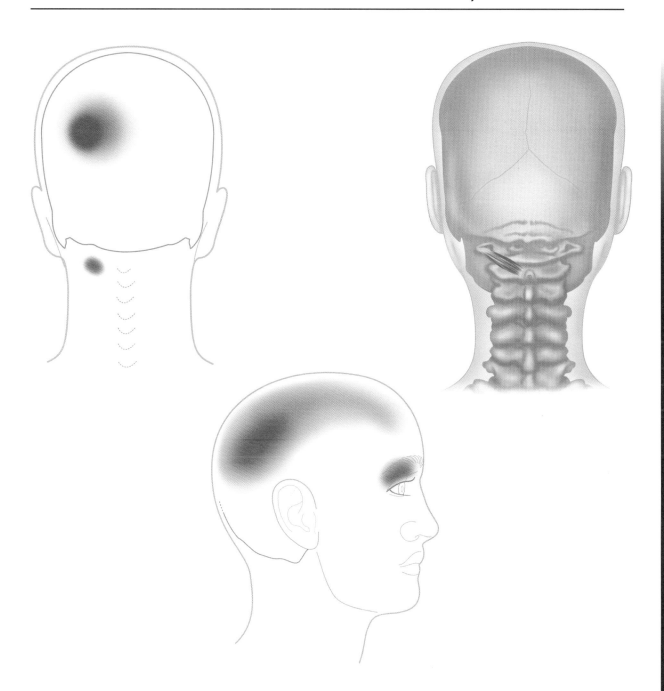

Muscle name
Obliquus capitis inferior.

Latin, *obliquus*, inclined, slanting; *capitis*, of the head; *inferior*, below.

Origin
Spinous process of axis (C2).

Insertion
Lateral mass of atlas (C1).

Action
Rotates atlanto-axial joint.

Kinetic chain comment
Any small change in head position will ultimately affect the status of this muscle.

Trigger point comment
Pain shooting from the back of the head into the eye is a regular complaint of headache, particularly migraine sufferers. As this is the pain referral of obliquus capitis inferior it should be included as part of any treatment plan for patients complaining of similar patterns.

Nerve
Suboccipital nerve (posterior primary ramus of C1).

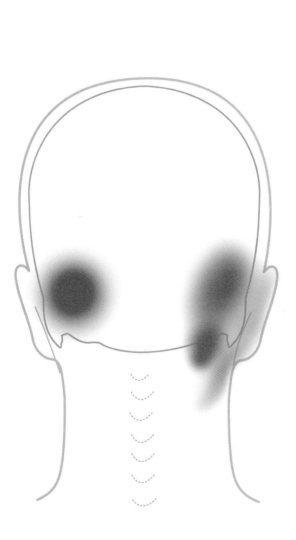

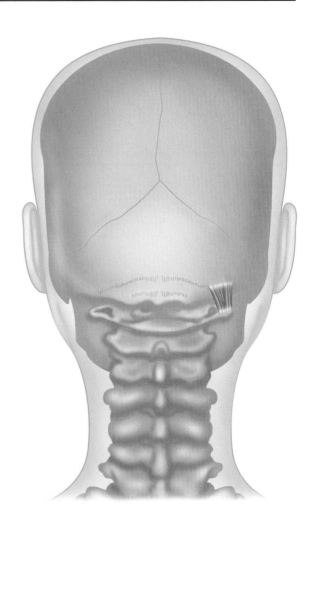

Muscle name
Obliquus capitis superior.

Latin, *obliquus*, inclined, slanting; *capitis*, of the head; *superior*, above.

Origin
Lateral mass of transverse process of atlas (C1).

Insertion
Lateral half of inferior nuchal line.

Action
Laterally flexes atlanto-occipital joint.

Kinetic chain comment
Decelerates flexion and contralateral extension of the head at the neck. Enriched with muscle spindles, the positioning of obliquus capitis superior and inferior is so important to efficient posture.

Trigger point comment
This muscle will cause dull, deep pain over the lateral aspects of the occipital bone with diffuse pain radiating down the sides of the jaw bone and into the ears.

Nerve
Suboccipital nerve (dorsal ramus of first cervical nerve, C1).

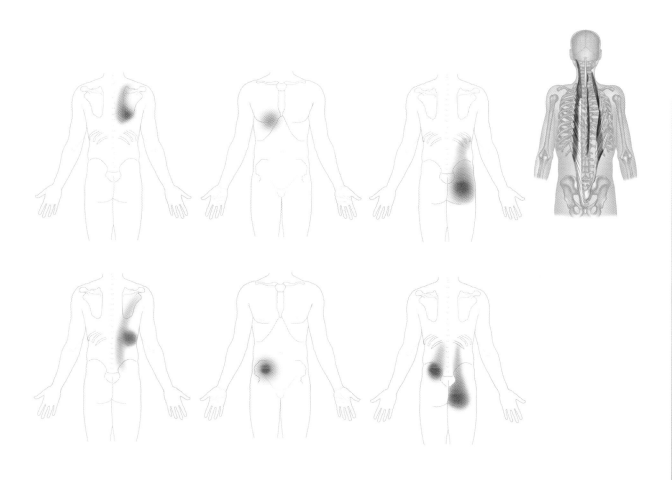

Muscle group
Erector spinae.

Latin, *sacrum*, sacred; *spinalis*, spinal.

Origin
All of the many erector spinae muscles conjoin the thoraco-lumbar fascia attaching at several different angles to the crest of the ilium and sacrum, spinous processes of the lumbar, and eleventh and twelfth thoracic vertebrae.

Insertion
Many varied attachments to the posterior costal bones, spinous and transverse processes of the thoracic and cervical vertebrae, and mastoid process of the temporal bone.

Action
Extends the vertebral column while the deep rotators and multifidi erectors rotate the column to the opposite side. The semispinalis extends the vertebral column and the head.

Kinetic chain comment
This group includes the iliocostalis, longissimus, spinalis, and multifidi. Eccentrically these muscles decelerate forward flexion, lateral flexion, and rotation. These muscles are the main stabilizers of the lumbar spine in the normal gait of movement.

Trigger point comment
These muscles can refer pain into the gluteal and sacral areas from the lumbar erectors. As a loose rule, pain generally refers up and out with trigger points in the suboccipitals, causing severe headaches, while mid-thoracic trigger points can refer pain into the anterior chest wall and abdomen. Pain experienced as rib pain can often be trigger point related. Trigger points in the cervical spine are often due to repeated supine sit-ups or crunches performed on the floor without first stabilizing the hyoid by means of correct tongue position. These in turn can perpetuate trigger points in the psoas, scalenes, sternocleidomastoideus and down the chain into the plantars.

Nerve
Dorsal rami of cervical, thoracic, and lumbar spinal nerves.

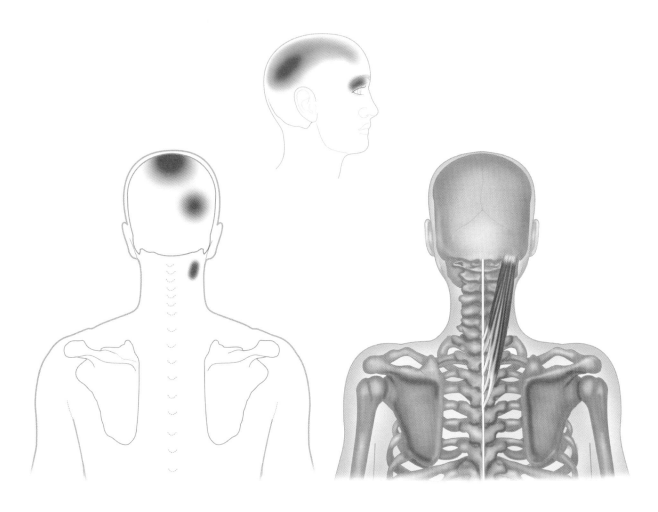

Muscle name

Splenius capitis.

Greek, *splenion*, bandage; **Latin**, *capitis*, of the head.

Origin

Inferior aspect of ligamentum nuchae. Spinous processes of C7 and T1–4.

Insertion

Mastoid process (posterior portion).

Action

Bilaterally extends the head and neck. Ipsilateral neck flexion and rotation.

Kinetic chain comment

Poor computer positioning or poor posture when reading can lead to stress of the splenius capitis. Eyes below the level of a computer screen require the operator to look up activating these muscles and over time creating a hyperextended cervical spine. This requires the pelvis to tilt anteriorly to flex the head so that the eyes can once again be level.

Trigger point comment

All the muscles of the posterior cervical spine should be investigated when patients complain of tension type headaches. This muscle is yet another contributor referring pain into the skull. Any head movement will involve splenius capitis in one of a number of ways and so this muscle is important to ensure appropriate head positioning. Pain spreads up to the crown of the head and into the back of the ipsilateral eye (similar to sternocleidomastoideus). Blurred vision and a headache with explosive pressure in the eye is often reported. Once serious eye pathologies have been ruled out, trigger points are the most likely cause of complaint.

Nerve

Dorsal rami of middle and lower cervical nerves.

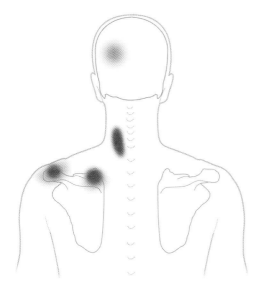

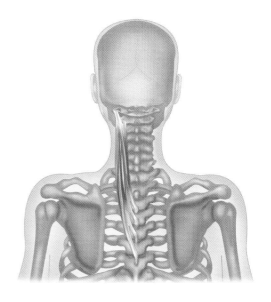

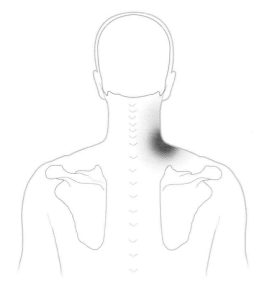

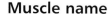

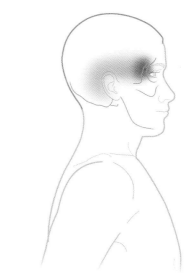

Kinetic chain comment
The cervical muscles, including splenius cervicis are as important to full body movement as the core musculature. Short splenius cervicis can displace the cervical or thoracic vertebrae affecting fourth layer muscles (splenii, semispinalis, multifidis, and rotatores) and positioning of thoracic ribs. Such changes result in postural adaptations up and down the kinetic chain.

Trigger point comment
Referred pain down onto the superior angle of the scapula and anteriorly out to the acromion process. Contributes to tension type headaches with pain felt over the temporal and occipital bones.

Nerve
Dorsal rami of spinal nerves.

Muscle name
Splenius cervicis.

Greek, *splenion*, bandage; **Latin**, *cervix*, neck.

Origin
Ligamentum nuchae. Spinous process of seventh cervical vertebra.

Insertion
Spinous process of C2 (axis).

Action
Extends the vertebral column. Keeps the spine upright, giving lift when standing.

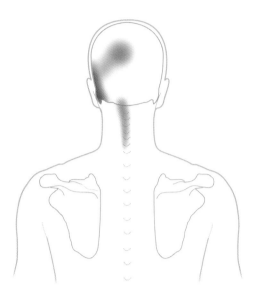

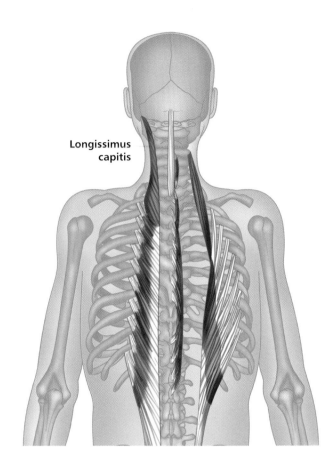

Longissimus capitis

Muscle name
Longissimus capitis.

Latin, *longissimus*, longest; *capitis*, of the head.

Origin
Upper five transverse processes of the thoracic vertebrae and articular processes of the fifth to seventh cervical vertebrae.

Insertion
Posterior margin of the mastoid process.

Action
This deep neck muscle extends the head and rotates the face toward the ipsilateral side.

Kinetic chain comment
Due to its close proximity with important neurovascular structures, this is an ideal muscle to use as an example of the need for differential diagnosis and the necessity to work within a multi-disciplinary context, referring when in any doubt. Pain, referred or otherwise in this area could be as a result of the following; degenerative disc disease, (segmental, subluxation, somatic dysfunction), C2/C3 radiculopathy, (bulging, prolapsed, herniated disc), fibromyalgia, osteoporosis,

osteoarthritis, rheumatoid arthritis, intervertebral or vertebral stenosis, vertebral vascular disorder, cerebral aneurysm, cerebral neoplasm (brain cancer), military neck (absence of normal cervical spine lordosis), cervical spine hyperlordosis, thoracic spine hyperkyphosis, scoliosis, tension/cluster headaches, suboccipital articular dysfunction, mastoiditis, cervical arthritis, cervical syndrome, subacute meningitis, polymyalgia rheumatica, polymyositis, systemic lupus erythematosus, acceleration/deceleration injury (whiplash), eye strain, ocular disease, sinusitis, tetanus, systemic infections or inflammation, nutritional inadequacy, metabolic imbalance, toxicity, side effects of medications. Appropriate screening will provide you with the information needed to know when to refer. Remember if in doubt, refer.

Trigger point comment
Pain referred from this muscle travels to the posterior aspect of the ear. The pain can also extend somewhat across the neck and behind the eyes. A contributor to headache pain with tenderness reported at the occipital bone and upper neck sometimes accompanied by numbness and tingling in the scalp.

Nerve
Dorsal rami of middle and lower cervical nerves.

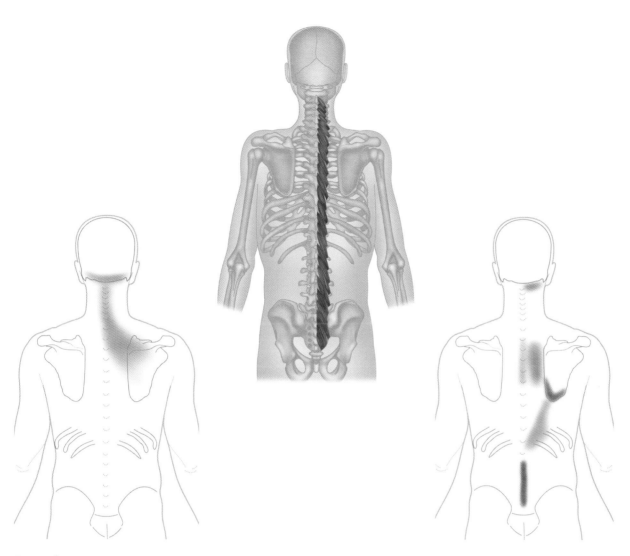

Muscle name
Multifidis.

Latin, *multi*, many, much; *findere*, to split.

Origin
Attaches to the posterior aspect of the iliac crest and sacrum, sacroiliac ligament, mamillary process of the lumbar vertebrae and the transverse processes of the thoracic vertebrae, including the articular processes of C4, 5, 6, and 7.

Insertion
Spinous processes of the superior vertebrae.

Action
Extends, laterally flexes, and rotates the vertebral column, in addition to extending and laterally rotating the pelvis. A core fourth layer muscle.

Kinetic chain comment
A major muscle in neuromuscular efficiency of the 'core'. The deep multifidus has a role in controlling intersegmental motion.

N.B. SPINAL INTEGRITY RELIES ON THE COMBINED ABILITY OF THE TRANSVERSUS ABDOMINIS MUSCLE TO MAINTAIN PELVIC STABILITY AND THE ACTION OF MULTIFIDIS AND ROTATORES TO STABILIZE THE SPINAL STRUCTURE.

Trigger point comment
Pain is reported at the spinous processes of L1–L5 and anteriorly to the abdomen. S1 projects pain down to the coccyx; this referral radiates laterally from the level of T4–T5 to the inferior angle of the scapula. Trigger points located in the cervical region of the multifidus refer pain from the suboccipital region referring down the posterior neck to the approximate segmental level of T3 and laterally to the rhomboids. There is also a lateral distribution at the base of the neck and upper back region.

Nerve
Dorsal rami of spinal nerves.

Muscles of the Trunk

Muscles of the Trunk

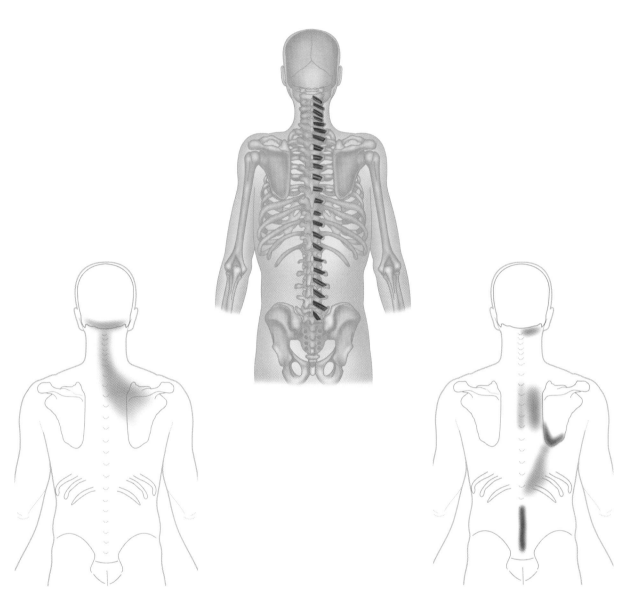

Muscle name
Rotatores.

Latin, *rot*, wheel.

Origin
(11 pairs from the sacrum to C2). Transverse process (inferior).

Insertion
Spinous process (superior).

Action
Extends and rotates the vertebrae.

Kinetic chain comment
A major muscle in neuromuscular efficiency of the 'core'.

N.B. SPINAL INTEGRITY RELIES ON THE COMBINED ABILITY OF THE TRANSVERSUS ABDOMINIS MUSCLE TO MAINTAIN PELVIC STABILITY AND THE ACTION OF MULTIFIDIS AND ROTATORES TO STABILIZE THE SPINAL STRUCTURE. DECELERATES FLEXION AND CONTRALATERAL ROTATION.

Trigger point comment
In my years of human cadaver studies, I have seen no need to separate the rotatores from the multifidi when dealing with MtPs. These muscles (I view them as one!) are basal skull pain generators as well as neck and scapular pain generators. Referral to a dry needle expert may be called for as these fourth layer muscles are difficult to treat with fingers and thumbs without many years experience.

Nerve
Posterior rami of the thoracic nerves.

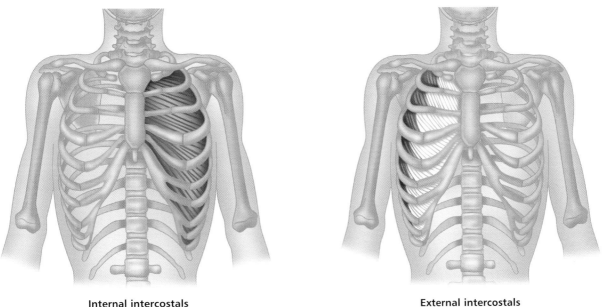

Internal intercostals   External intercostals

Muscles of the Trunk

Muscle name
Intercostales (externi, interni).

Latin, *inter*, between; costal, rib; *externi*, external; *interni*, internal.

Origin
Inferior border of ribs as far back as posterior angles.

Insertion
Superior border of ribs below, passing obliquely downwards and backwards.

Action
Fix intercostal spaces during respiration. Aids forced inspiration by elevating ribs.

Kinetic chain comment
These are the principle muscles of respiration. Problems with these muscles can literally change the internal pH of the body. The intercostals draw the central tendon downward during resting respiration. These muscles will also affect frontal plane movement along the lateral line.

Trigger point comment
Difficulty in breathing with sharp pain felt on exhaling in particular. Exercise or activity induced breathing difficulties can lead to trigger points being mistaken for exercise induced asthma.

Nerve
Muscular collateral branches of intercostal nerves.

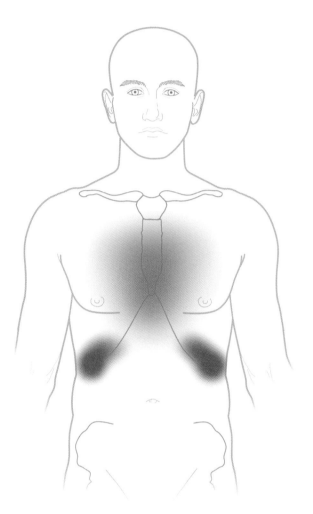

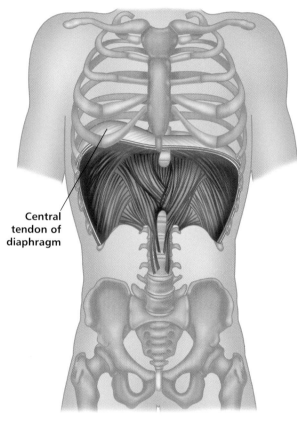

Central tendon of diaphragm

Muscle name
Diaphragm.

Greek, *partition*, wall.

Origin
Sternal portion: Two slips from posterior aspect of xiphoid process.
Costal portion: Medial and lateral arcuate ligaments, inner aspect of the lower six ribs.
Lumbar portion: Crura from bodies of L1, 2 (left), L1–3 (right).

Insertion
Central tendon.

Action
Inspiration and assists in raising intra-abdominal pressure.

Kinetic chain comment
This dome-shaped musculofibrous muscle is penetrated by the aorta, vena cava and the oesophagus. Fascial investments with the quadratus lumborum and psoas muscles highlight the importance of this structure, linking as it does the lower and upper quarters. Psoas and quadratus lumborum should be treated along with the diaphragm when dealing with respiratory dysfunction.

Trigger point comment
Patients complain of chest pain, dyspnoea, and not being able to take a full functional breath. A stitch in the side is common. Sudden increases in exercise intensity or physical activities can activate, or be the cause of trigger point formation in the diaphragm.

Nerve
Phrenic nerve (ventral rami), C3–C5.

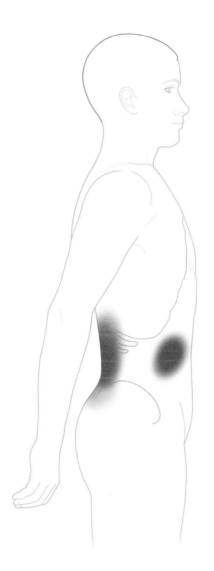

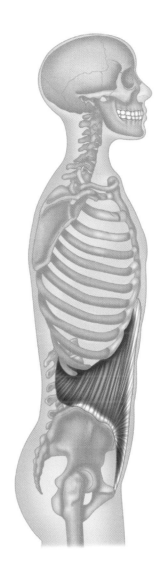

Muscle name
Obliquus internus abdominis.

Latin, *obliquus*, inclined, slanting; *internus*, internal; *abdominis*, belly / stomach.

Origin
Lumbar fascia, anterior two-thirds of iliac crest and lateral two-thirds of inguinal ligament.

Insertion
Costal margin, aponeurosis of rectus sheath (anterior and posterior), conjoint tendon to pubic crest and pectineal line.

Action
Supports abdominal wall, assists forced respiration, aids raising intra-abdominal pressure and, with muscles of other side, abducts and rotates trunk. Conjoint tendon supports posterior wall of inguinal canal.

Kinetic chain comment
The most common mistake in exercise programs is the attempt to isolate the internal obliques in relation to the other abdominal muscles, excluding efforts to train this muscle in the functional manner in which it operates. The internal obliques typically becomes inhibited when stressed, leading to muscular compensations and change in pelvic positioning.

Trigger point comment
Any abdominal pain should be treated with caution. Any suspicion concerning the type of pain or symptoms should be the cue for referral to a doctor. Internal obliques trigger points refer pain in many directions in the abdomen, including the lower back. Pain across the midline is possible. Patients complain of burning, bloatedness and stomach swelling.

Nerve
Ventral rami of thoracic nerves, T7–T12, ilioinguinal and iliohypogastric nerves.

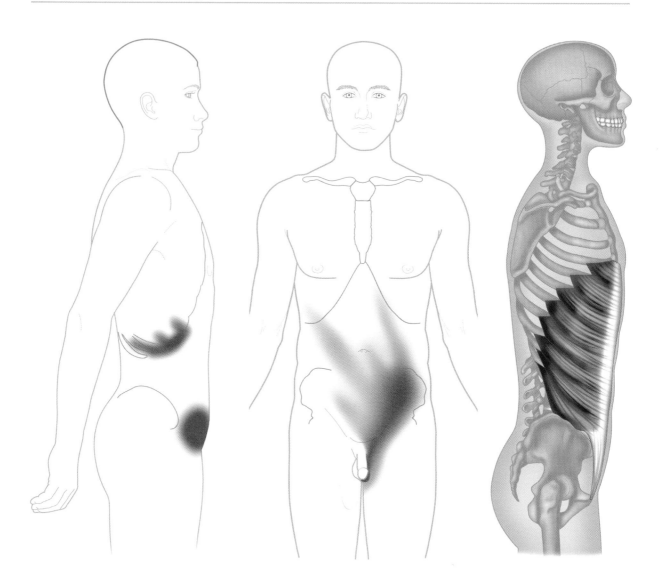

Muscle name
Obliquus externus abdominis.

Latin, *obliquus*, inclined, slanting; *externus*, external; *abdominis*, belly / stomach.

Origin
Anterior angles of lower eight ribs.

Insertion
Outer anterior half of iliac crest, inguinal ligament, pubic tubercle and crest, and aponeurosis of anterior rectus sheath.

Action
Supports abdominal wall, assists forced expiration, aids raising intra-abdominal pressure and, with muscles of opposite side, abducts and rotates trunk.

Kinetic chain comment
When considering physical activities to improve the function of the external obliques, one should try to include both open and closed kinetic chain movements. The feet should be placed on and taken off the floor. Movements such as those seen during swimming involve the external obliques in a way that can be trained with dry training but requires imagination.

Trigger point comment
Pain can refer down into the groin and sometimes to the testicles. Similar to the other abdominal muscles, external obliques trigger points can refer pain anywhere locally throughout the abdominal region. This pain is often exacerbated during the menstrual cycle.

Nerve
Ventral rami of thoracic nerves, T5–T12.

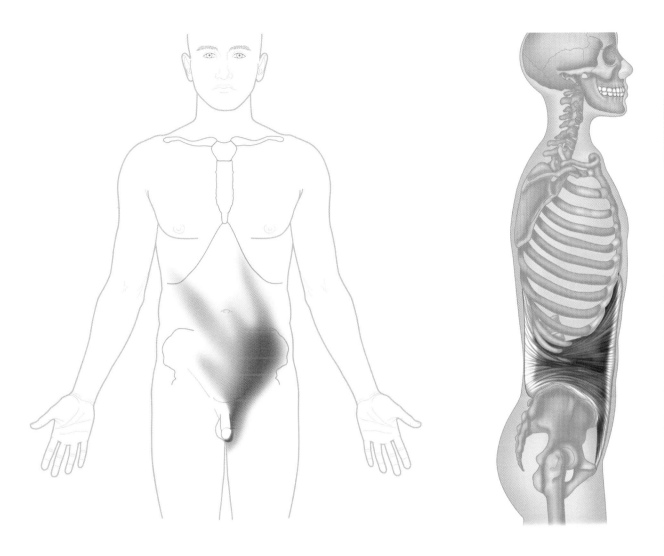

Muscle name
Transversus abdominis.

Latin, *transversus*, across, crosswise; *abdominis*, belly / stomach.

Origin
Costal margin, lumbar fascia, anterior two-thirds of iliac crest, and lateral half of inguinal ligament.

Insertion
Aponeurosis of posterior and anterior rectus sheath and conjoint tendon to pubic crest and pectineal line.

Action
Supports abdominal wall, aids forced expiration, and raising intra-abdominal pressure. Conjoint tendon supports posterior wall of inguinal canal.

Kinetic chain comment
All abdominal muscles work moment to moment as we move, providing the tension required to translate forces from the lower limbs to the upper limbs. Transversus abdominis is the deepest of these muscles and each one (right and left) wraps up the organs horizontally. Transversus abdominis fascial attachments include the lumbar vertebrae, rib cage, iliac crest, and inguinal ligament. It also connects directly into the linea alba providing a link between the xiphoid process, pyramidalis, and the pubic bone. Transversus abdominis therefore provides essential support for the internal organs, and provides tensional support and lift for the L2, L3 lumbar vertebrae.

Trigger point comment
Pain is experienced across the upper abdomen with a focus on the xiphoid process. Patients can also experience a marked enthesitis along the inferior costal margin. Coughing is especially distressing.

Nerve
Ventral rami of thoracic nerves, T7–T12, ilioinguinal and iliohypogastric nerves.

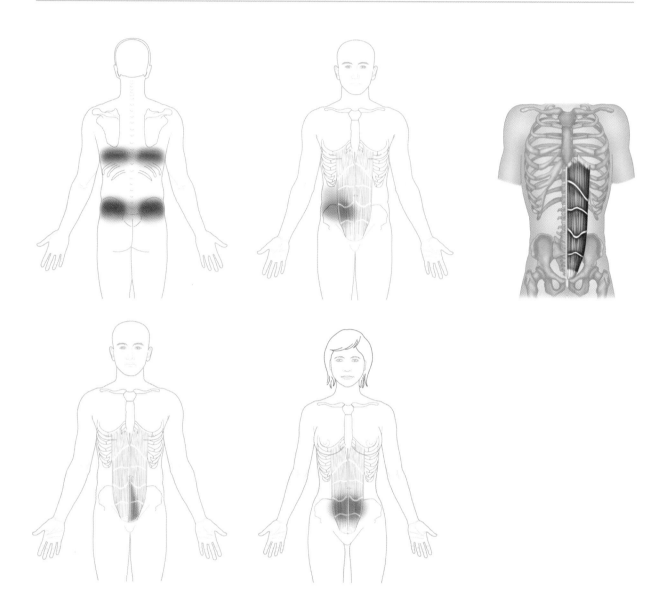

Muscle name
Rectus abdominis.

Latin, *rectum*, straight; *abdominis*, belly / stomach.

Origin
Pubic crest and symphysis pubis via two tendons separated by the linea alba.

Insertion
Costal cartilages of the fifth to seventh ribs and xiphoid process.

Action
With the origin fixed, the chest wall will move towards the pelvis. With the insertion fixed, the pelvis will move towards the chest.

Kinetic chain comment
This muscle decelerates trunk extension through eccentric action. It is worth noting that this range of motion cannot be achieved with conventional sit-ups completed on the floor, which can contribute to muscle imbalances and neuromuscular inefficiency of the core.

Trigger point comment
Rectus abdominis has two distinct pain patterns; one at the level of the xiphoid process, spreading bilaterally across the midback, and the second at the level between the umbilicus and the inguinal ligament spreading pain into the sacroiliac and low back. Rectus abdominis trigger points can also cause chest pain, heartburn, belching, and can cause diarrhea, dysmenorrhea and appendicitis (McBurney's point).

Nerve
Ventral rami of thoracic nerves, T5–T12.

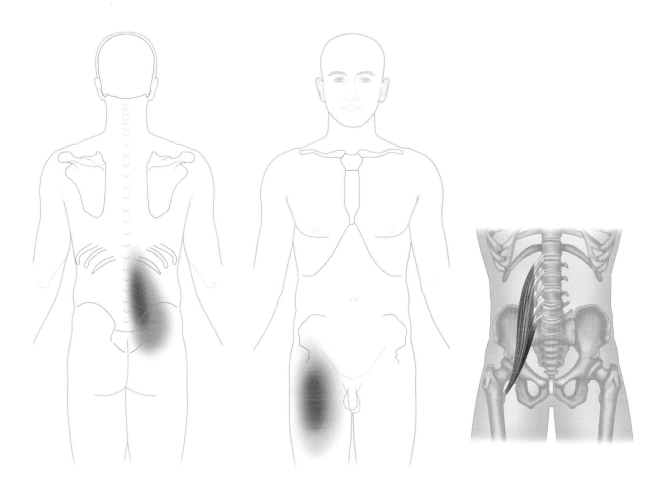

Muscle name
Psoas major.

Greek, *psoas*, muscle of the loin; *major*, large.

Origin
Transverse processes of L1–L5, bodies of T12–L5, and intervertebral discs below bodies of T12–L4.

Insertion
Middle surface of lesser trochanter of femur.

Action
Flexes and medially rotates the hip.

Kinetic chain comment
Psoas major eccentrically decelerates hip extension and external rotation at the hip. This muscle is typically short, causing inhibition in the gluteals. This sets up the foundation for kinetic chain neuromuscular changes and the formation of trigger points.

Trigger point comment
Prolonged sitting has been identified as a significant precursor to the formation of trigger points. Trigger points form in psoas major as a result of primary trigger points in related muscles of the psoas functional unit. These include rectus femoris, pectineus, sartorius, tensor fascia latae, the adductors (longus, brevis, magnus), and gracilis. Pain is felt as a vertical pattern ipsilaterally along the lumbar spine, and downward over the sacroiliac joint and gluteal region. Pain can also be present in the groin and medial thigh. Psoas pain can be mistaken for lumbago and disc pathology.

Nerve
Ventral rami of lumbar nerves, L1–L4.

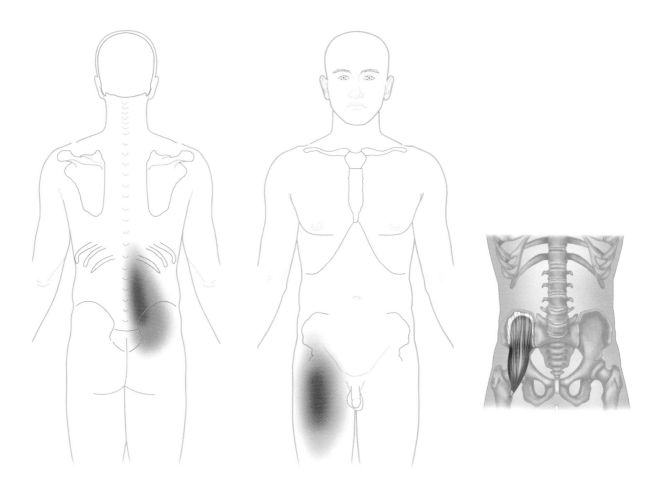

Muscle name
Iliacus.

Latin, pertaining to the loin.

Origin
Iliac fossa by means of the superior two-thirds of the crest of the ilium, iliolumbar, and anterior sacroiliac ligament and ala of the sacrum.

Insertion
Blending with the lateral aspect of the psoas major over the pelvic rim, slightly distal to the lesser trochanter of the femur and a few fibres merging with the joint capsule of the hip.

Action
With the origin fixed, it will draw the femur forwards in hip flexion, adduction, and internal rotation. With the insertion fixed and acting bilaterally, the pelvis is drawn forward tilting the pelvis with flexion at the hip but with the trunk moving increasing lumbar lordosis.

Unilaterally, iliacus will assist in lateral flexion of the trunk toward the same side.

Kinetic chain comment
The iliacus and psoas major (including psoas minor if one is evident) work together to provide a deceleration of internal rotation of the femur on heel strike and slow hip extension. Bilateral contraction of this fleshy triangular muscle provides stability to the lumbar spine. These muscles are rich in muscle spindles and are therefore prone to shorten under stress. This in turn provides inhibition to the gluteus maximus.

Trigger point comment
Trigger points can form in the gastor of iliacus and its associated muscles psoas major/minor, referring pain across the lower back, down into the buttock, anterior thigh, and groin. Difficulty in breathing and urinating are often reported.

Nerve
Femoral nerve, L2–L4.

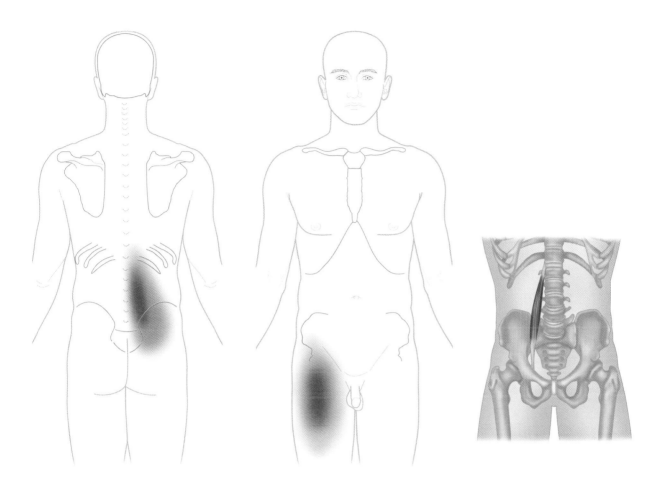

Muscle name
Psoas minor.

Greek, *psoas*, muscle of the loin; *minor*, small.

Origin
Bodies of T12 and L1 and intervening intervertebral disc.

Insertion
Fascia over psoas major and iliacus.

Action
Weak flexor of trunk.

Kinetic chain comment
This muscle is present in only 50–60% of the population. Due to its unique relationship connecting the upper body and lower limb, problems in this muscle result in full body kinetic chain adaptations and distortions. These can include neck, lower back, knee, and foot pain.

Trigger point comment
Posterior tilted pelvis can be a symptom of trigger points in this muscle. This causes a flat back posture and compressed intervertebral discs. Low back pain is the classical referral pattern, but pain can also be referred into the groin and thigh.

Nerve
Anterior primary rami of L1, 2.

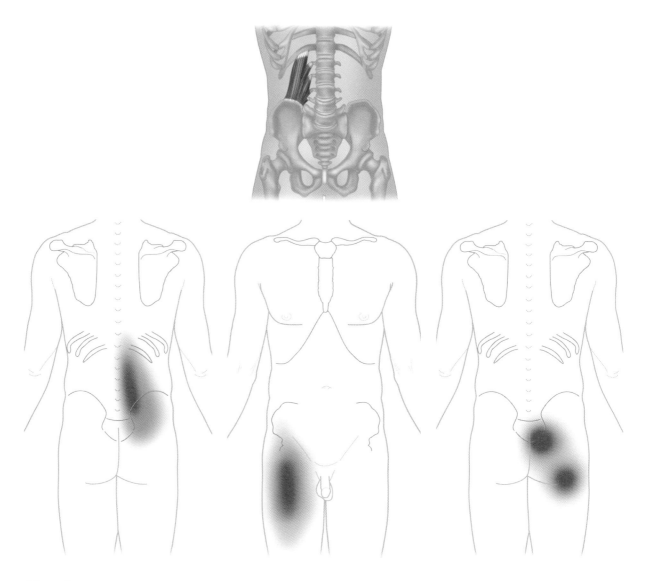

Muscle name
Quadratus lumborum.

Latin, *quadratus*, squared; *lumbar*, loin.

Origin
Inferior border of twelfth rib.

Insertion
Apices of transverse processes of L1–L4, iliolumbar ligament, and posterior third of iliac crest.

Action
Fixes twelfth rib during respiration and laterally flexes trunk.

Kinetic chain comment
Short quadratus lumborum leads to a functional short leg on the same side. This in turn leads to muscle adaptations, whereby the contralateral adductors may shorten in an effort to pull the femur more posteriorly into the acetabulum. This can create the look of a short leg on the contralateral side and cause subluxation at the pubic symphysis and sacroiliac joint. Kinetic chain problems continue both up and down the chain.

Trigger point comment
Pain is experienced at the sacroiliac joint and into the gluteals and hip. Referred pain in the anterior thigh and groin can be very painful. Fear of coughing or sneezing due to intolerable pain in the lower back is common. Difficulty sleeping on the affected side due to pain. Trigger points in the quadratus lumborum can cause the hip to hike and lead to a scoliosis and subsequent anatomical short leg.

Nerve
Ventral rami of the subcostal nerve and upper three or four lumbar nerves, T12, L1–3.

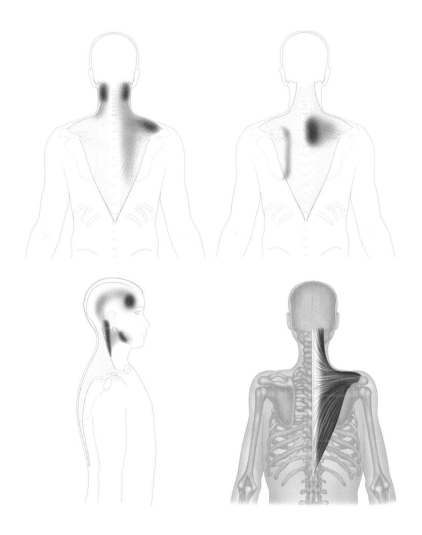

Muscle name
Trapezius.

Latin, *trapezoides*, table shaped.

Origin
Medial third superior nuchal line, ligament nuchae, spinous processes and supraspinous ligaments to T12.

Insertion
Upper fibres to lateral third of posterior border of clavicle; lower fibres to medial acromion, and superior lip of spine of scapula to deltoid tubercle.

Action
Laterally rotates, elevates, and retracts scapula. If scapula is fixed, extends and laterally flexes neck.

Kinetic chain comment
As this muscle is an important neck muscle, any spastic activity in the sternocleidomastoideus, suboccipitals, scalenes, longus colli, levator scapulae, or many other muscles will have an effect on the status of trapezius. Many people hold emotional tension in the upper trapezius. Trapezius decelerates the head (upper portion) while the middle portion decelerates protraction. The lower portion decelerates shoulder elevation.

Trigger point comment
Trigger points here lead to tension headaches with sharp pain felt in the temporal bone and into the masseter, behind the eye and ear (on the same side), and along the side of the neck. Occasionally, pain will travel to the back of the head and a burning pain down into the vertebral side of the scapula and midback. Trapezius trigger points can cause loss of balance and dizziness. Trigger points in this muscle are often mistaken for disc pathologies, neuralgia, spinal stenosis, shoulder bursitis, or arthritis.

Nerve
Motor supply: Accessory XI nerve.
Sensory supply (proprioception): Ventral ramus of cervical nerves, C2–C4.

Muscles of the Shoulder, Arm, and Hand

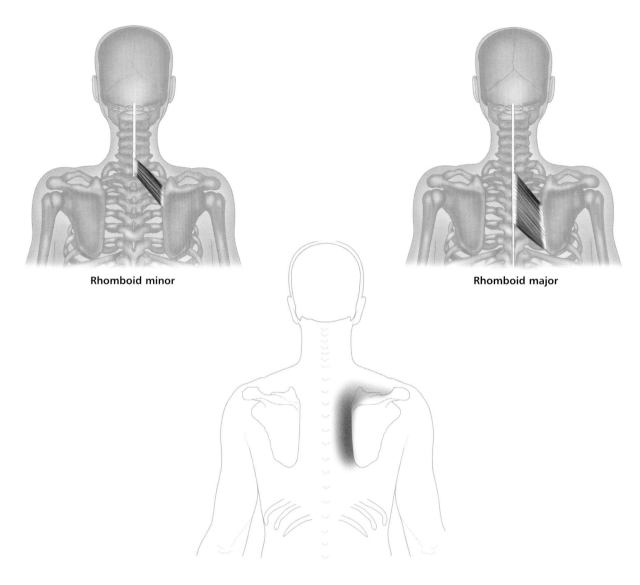

Rhomboid minor   Rhomboid major

Muscles of the Shoulder, Arm, and Hand

Muscle name
Rhomboids.

Greek, *rhomb*, a parallelogram with oblique angles and only the opposite sides equal; *minor*, small; *major*, large.

Origin
Spines of C7–T5 and supraspinous ligaments.

Insertion
Lower half of posteromedial border of scapula, from the root of the inferior angle to upper part of triangular area at base of scapular spine.

Action
Retracts the scapula. Adducts, elevates, and internally rotates the scapula.

Kinetic chain comment
A hypertonic rhomboid will have a marked effect on the positioning of the scapula by lifting and retracting it. This in turn will inhibit the neural status of the serratus anterior, in turn affecting external oblique and so on along the chain. Force couple actions will be out of sequence, setting up the ideal environment for strain and overuse injury. When serratus anterior is hypertonic, the rhomboids become inhibited and the scapula will sit wide and drop.

Trigger point comment
Pain is experienced around the vertebral border of the scapula and especially at night when at rest. The scalenes are primary sponsors of referred pain in this area and are worth treating when patients present with this pain pattern.

Nerve
Dorsal scapular nerve, C4, 5.

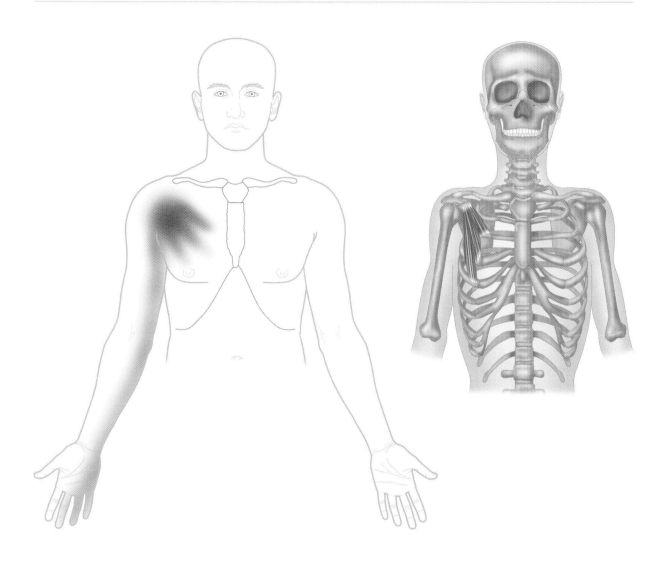

Muscle name
Pectoralis minor.

Latin, *pectoralis*, chest; *minor*, small.

Origin
Third, fourth, and fifth ribs.

Insertion
Medial and upper surface of the coracoid process of scapula.

Action
Elevates ribs if scapula is fixed, protracts scapula (assists serratus anterior) and stiffens to support abduction and flexion at the shoulder joint.

Kinetic chain comment
Pectoralis minor provides the tension to protract the scapula against the posterior rib cage, providing a relationship with the axial skeleton so that some movement can efficiently occur at the glenohumeral joint (e.g. lateral arm raise).

Trigger point comment
Anterior chest pain with referred pain down the medial side of the arm and extending into the third, fourth, and fifth fingers. This pain can be mistaken for signs of heart disease. Most often mistaken for carpal tunnel syndrome due to restricted blood vessels and compressed nerves. Often a part of a double crush (scalenes) or treble crush problem where all muscles must be cleared of trigger points before homeostasis is restored.

Nerve
Medial pectoral nerve, C7, 8, T1.

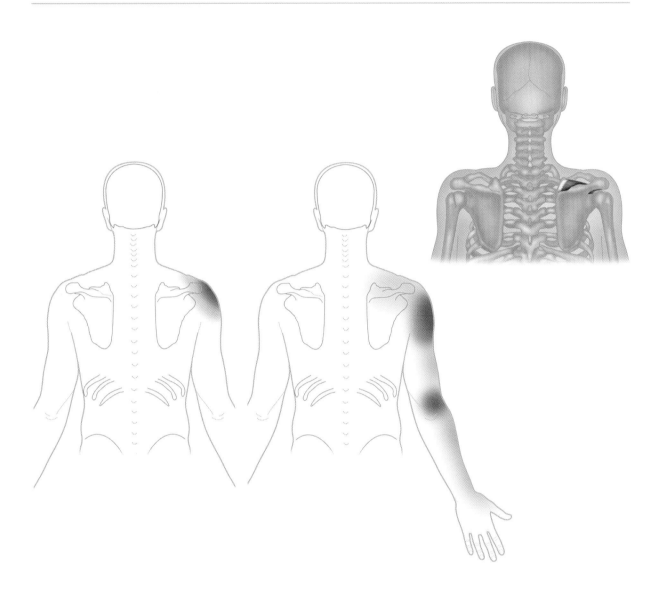

Muscle name
Supraspinatus.

Latin, *supra*, above; *spina*, spine.

Origin
Medial three quarters of supraspinous fossa of scapula, upper surface of spine (bipennate).

Insertion
Superior facet on greater tuberosity of humerus and capsule of shoulder joint.

Action
Abducts arm, weak external rotator, and stabilizes the glenohumeral joint.

Kinetic chain comment
Supraspinatus works in conjunction with the deltoid to produce abduction at the glenohumeral joint. Due to its insertion superiorly onto the greater tuberosity, it pulls the humeral head into the glenohumeral joint providing the stability needed for the deltoid, pulling halfway down the humerus to abduct the arm.

Trigger point comment
Deep pain in the lateral shoulder, forearm, and wrist. Radiating pain into the lateral epicondyle can lead to a misdiagnosis of tennis elbow, while the shoulder pain can be mistaken for bursitis. Difficulty combing your hair or raising the arm in flexion are signs of the presence of trigger points.

Nerve
Suprascapular nerve, C5, 6.

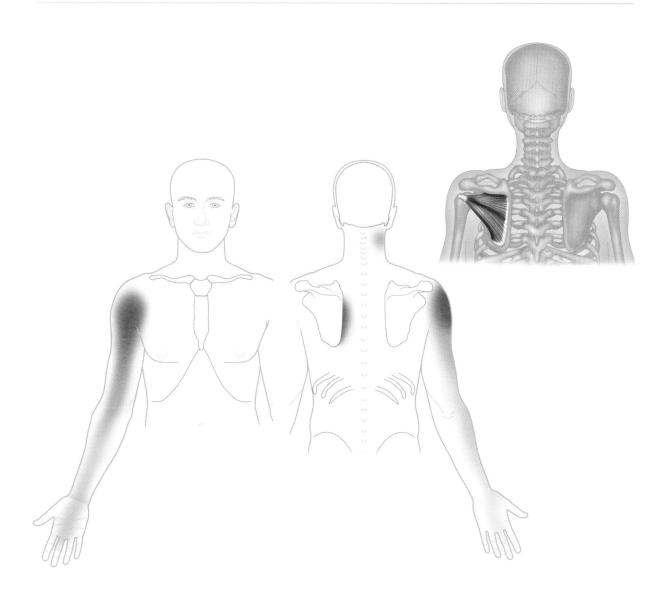

Muscle name
Infraspinatus.

Latin, *infra*, below; *spina*, spine.

Origin
Medial three quarters of infraspinous fossa of scapula and fibrous intermuscular septa.

Insertion
Middle facet of greater tuberosity of humerus and capsule of shoulder joint.

Action
Laterally rotates arm and stabilizes shoulder joint.

Kinetic chain comment
An important muscle in scapula positioning. Decelerates internal rotation and shoulder flexion. Like all the SITS muscles, infraspinatus relies on an efficient core (lumbo-pelvic-hip complex) to translate forces needed from the lower limbs to the upper limbs.

Trigger point comment
Deep shoulder joint pain also felt in the biceps brachii and down the side of the shoulder radiating as far as the thumb. Severe pain in the anterior deltoid and bicipital groove are a common aspect of these trigger points, with pain also experienced in the posterior neck. Combined with other SITS muscles, these trigger points can cause symptoms mistaken for adhesive capsulitis (frozen shoulder syndrome).

Nerve
Suprascapular nerve, C5, 6.

Muscles of the Shoulder, Arm, and Hand

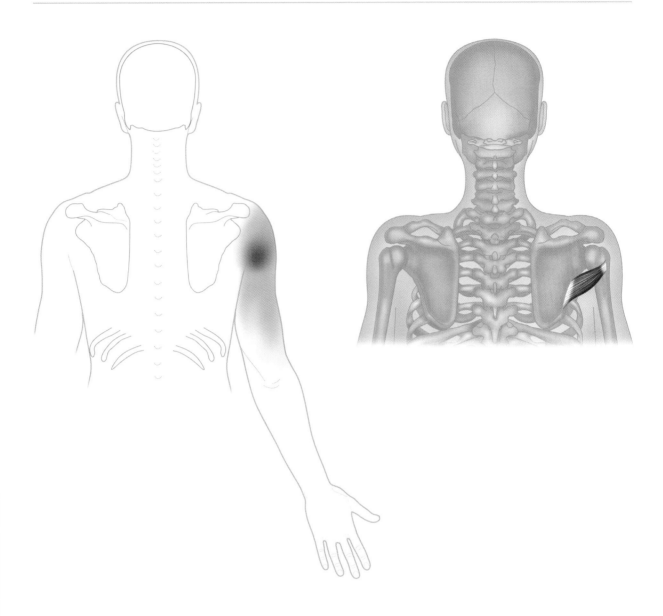

Muscle name
Teres minor.

Latin, *teres*, rounded, finely shaped; *minor*, small.

Origin
Middle third lateral border of scapula above teres major.

Insertion
Inferior facet of greater tuberosity of humerus (below infraspinatus) and capsule of shoulder joint.

Action
Laterally rotates arm and stabilizes shoulder joint.

Kinetic chain comment
Teres minor decelerates internal rotation of the shoulder joint. Inhibition of this muscle due to short/spastic subscapularis, latissimus dorsi, teres major, and the pectoralis major muscles sets up the ideal conditions for repetitive stress in sports such as swimming, rugby, and any activity involving acceleration through internal/external rotation and flexion/extension of the shoulder complex.

Trigger point comment
Numbness or tingling will be felt in the fourth and fifth fingers of the same arm as well as pain in the posterior shoulder at the greater tuberosity. Teres minor trigger points are often sponsored by subscapularis.

Nerve
Axillary nerve, C5, 6 (from posterior cord of the brachial plexus).

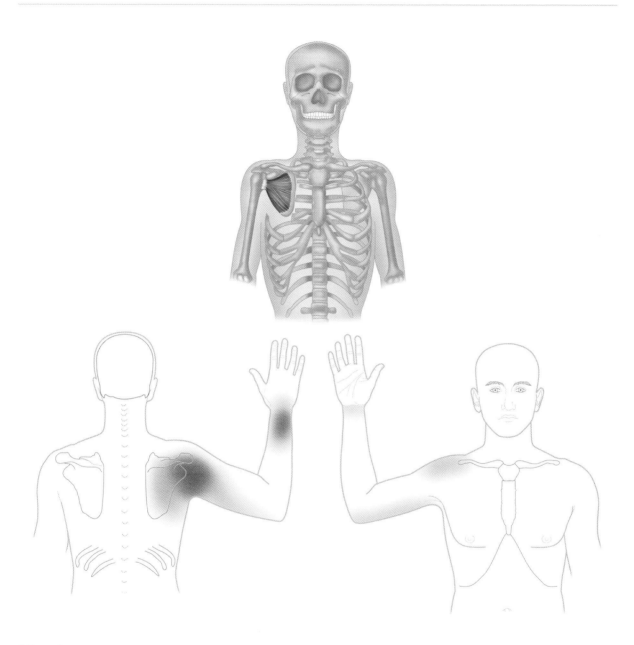

Muscle name
Subscapularis.

Latin, *sub*, under; *scapular*, pertaining to the scapula.

Origin
Medial two-thirds of subscapular fossa.

Insertion
Lesser tuberosity of humerus, upper medial lip of bicipital groove, capsule of shoulder joint.

Action
Medially rotates arm and stabilizes shoulder joint.

Kinetic chain comment
Eccentrically decelerates external rotation of the glenohumeral joint. This muscle has proved itself time and again to be worthy of special treatment focus in frozen shoulder and carpal tunnel syndrome complaints.

Trigger point comment
Deep pain felt in the posterior shoulder and wrist. Pain can radiate down the front of the arm. Spot tenderness on the lesser tuberosity of the humerus is common. Subscapularis trigger points are often mistaken for bursitis, adhesive capsulitis, bicipital tendonitis, arthritis, and rotator cuff injury. Pain and stiffness are a result of trigger points in the subscapularis.

Nerve
Upper and lower subscapular nerve, C5, 6 (from posterior cord of the brachial plexus).

Muscles of the Shoulder, Arm, and Hand

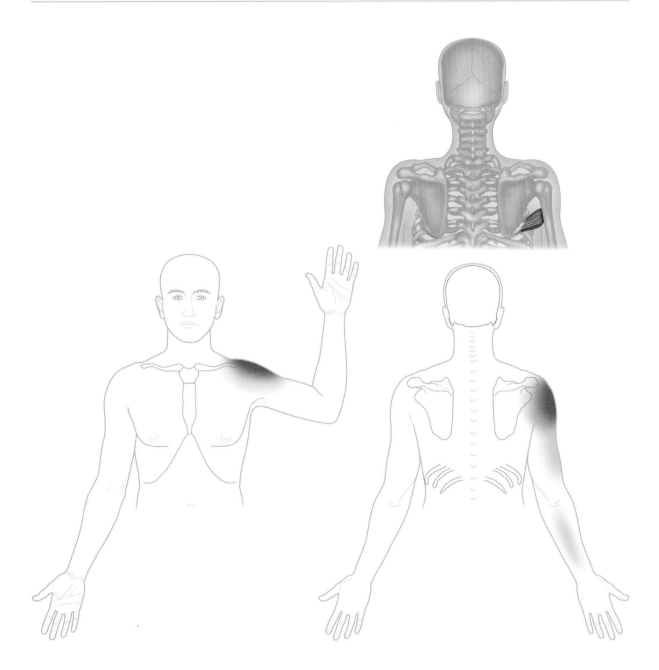

Muscle name
Teres major.

Latin, *teres*, rounded, finely shaped; *major*, large.

Origin
Arising from the dorsal humeral surface of the inferior angle of the scapula at the level of the lower third portion.

Insertion
Muscle fibres adhere to the fascia of latissimus dorsi, rising up to attach to the crest of the intertubercular groove.

Action
This muscle is affectionately known as *latissimus dorsi's* 'little helper'. It medially rotates, extends, and adducts the humerus at the glenohumeral joint.

Kinetic chain comment
This muscle helps to eccentrically decelerate flexion, abduction, and external rotation of the humerus.

Trigger point comment
Pain is experienced in the posterior deltoid.

Nerve
Lower subscapular nerve, C5–C7 (from posterior cord of the brachial plexus).

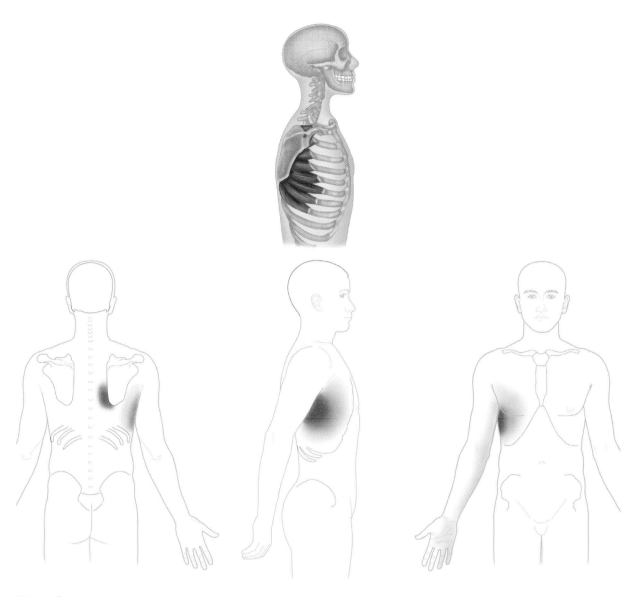

Muscle name
Serratus anterior.

Latin, *serratus*, serrated; *anterior*, before.

Origin
Upper eight ribs and anterior intercostal membranes from midclavicular line. Lower four interdigitating with external oblique.

Insertion
Inner medial border scapula. 1 and 2: upper angle; 3 and 4: length of costal surface; 5 to 8: inferior angle.

Action
Laterally rotates and protracts scapula.

Kinetic chain comment
Eccentrically decelerates adduction and medial rotation of the inferior angle of the scapula. Actions will change depending on the origin or insertion being fixed. With the arm static, movement occurs at the rib cage, accelerating or decelerating the ribs as required (e.g. forced exhalation).

Trigger point comment
Pain will be experienced on the side of the rib cage travelling into the armpit and posteriorly to the medial aspect of the inferior angle of the scapula. Pain is often mistaken for C8 nerve problems, as pain is referred down the inside of the arm into the palm, first (little), and second fingers. As this muscle has many digitations, careful assessment is required to locate active central trigger points.

Nerve
Long thoracic nerve, C5–C8 (from roots) slips from ribs 1 and 2: C5; 3 and 4: C6; 5 to 8: C7/8.

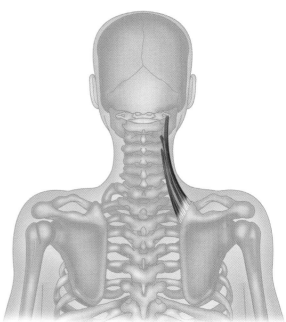

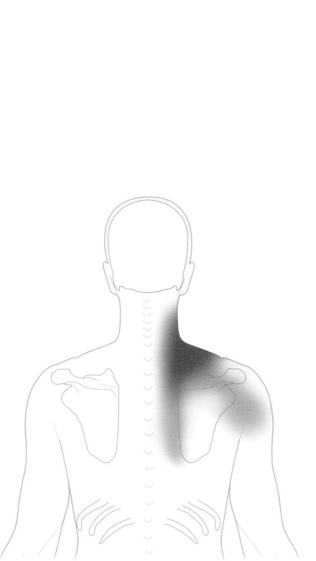

Muscle name

Levator scapulae.

Latin, *levare*, to lift; *scapulae*, shoulder, blade(s).

Origin

Posterior tubercles of transverse processes of C1–C4.

Insertion

Upper part of medial border of scapula.

Action

Elevates medial border of scapula.

Kinetic chain comment

Levator scapulae acts eccentrically to decelerate the downward forces created by the lower fibres of trapezius and serratus anterior. Levator scapulae decelerates contralateral side flexion in the cervical spine.

Trigger point comment

Almost all neck pain will have trigger point contribution and this muscle is commonly involved. Pain will be experienced at the angle of the neck from the superior angle making its way down to the medial aspect of the inferior angle with spillover all the way along the medial border of the scapula. Patients often report a stiff neck and reduced range of motion.

Nerve

Dorsal scapular nerve, C4, 5, and cervical nerve, C3, 4.

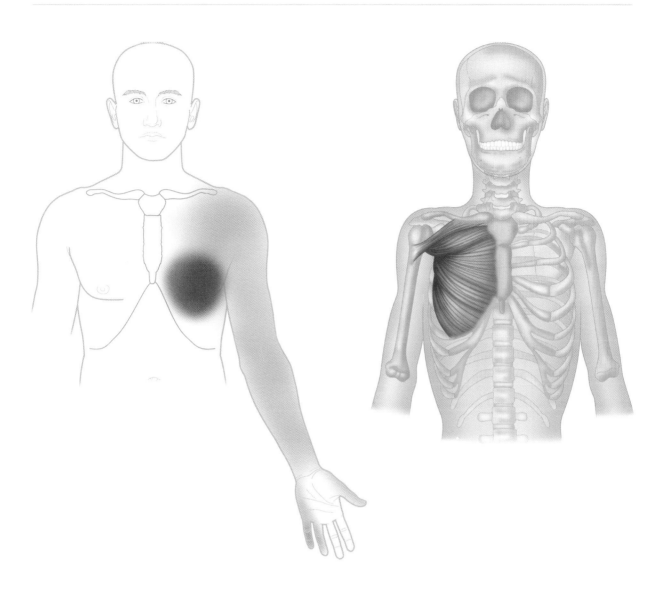

Muscle name
Pectoralis major.

Latin, *pectoralis*, chest; *major*, large.

Origin
Medial half of the anterior surface of the clavicle, anterior surface of the manubrium and sternum, and cartilage of the ribs (1–6).

Insertion
By means of a laminated tendon into the lateral crest of the intertubercular groove of the humerus.

Action
With the origin fixed, it will adduct and medially rotate the humerus. With the insertion fixed, it can assist in breathing (forced inspiration, as it elevates the chest). Assists in shoulder stabilization during overhead movements.

Kinetic chain comment
Eccentrically decelerates shoulder extension, horizontal abduction and external rotation and retraction of the shoulder joint.

Trigger point comment
This muscle can develop multiple trigger points due to its clavicular and sternal fibres firing pain across the anterior deltoid and down the lateral aspect of the arm into the thumb and fourth and fifth fingers. A rare trigger point can mimic symptoms of angina pectoris. Pain from these trigger points can also be felt as interscapular and subscapular pain. Restricted abduction will be evident.

Nerve
Medial nerve, C6–8, T1.

Muscles of the Shoulder, Arm, and Hand

Muscles of the Shoulder, Arm, and Hand

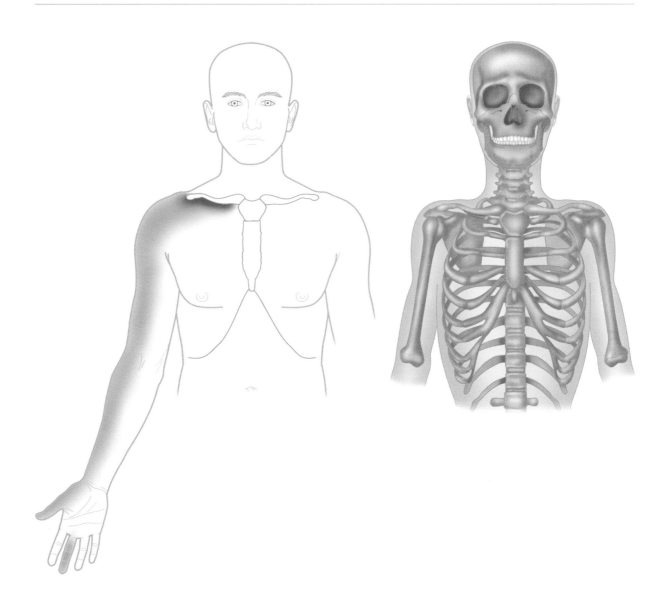

Muscle name
Subclavius.

Latin, *sub*, under; *clavis*, key, clavicle.

Origin
First rib about its junction of bone and costal cartilage.

Insertion
Undersurface of the clavicle to the subclavian groove.

Action
Pulling the clavicle towards the sternoclavicular joint.

Kinetic chain comment
Weak lumbo-pelvic-hip musculature can contribute to

the formation of trigger points in this muscle. Change in position of the scapula will compromise subclavius and lead to trigger point formation.

Trigger point comment
Pain is referred to the ipsilateral biceps brachii and lateral forearm. Locally pain will be experienced just below the clavicle and can be felt as pins and needles in the arm, shoulder, and hand. It typically bypasses the elbow and wrist, resulting in pain in the radial half of the hand, thumb, and middle finger.

Nerve
Nerve to subclavius, C5, 6.

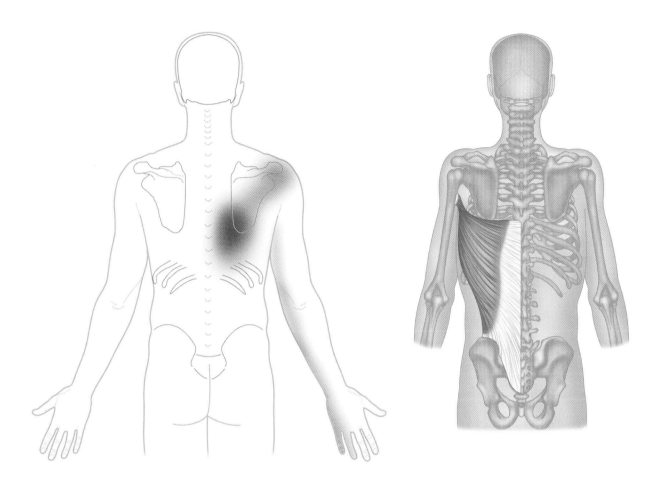

Muscle
Latissimus dorsi (LD).

Latin, *latissimus*, widest; *dorsi*, of the back.

Origin
Spinous processes of inferior six thoracic vertebrae, thoracolumbar fascia, iliac crest, and inferior three or four ribs.

Insertion
Intertubercular groove of the humerus.

Action
Along with its 'little helper' (*teres major*) this muscle adducts, extends, and medially rotates the humerus in the glenohumeral joint (GHJ).

Kinetic chain comment
A neuromuscular efficient core is required in order for the LD to provide the necessary forces to carry out some function at the GHJ. Neuromuscular inefficiency leads to the foundations for repetitive stress and associated 'frozen shoulder' type symptoms. LD decelerates lateral rotation, flexion, and abduction of the humerus in the GHJ.

When the insertion of LD is fixed, it plays a role in tilting of the pelvis in an anterolateral direction. A bilateral contraction leads to a hyperextension of the lower back with accompanying anterior tilting of the pelvis. Of course a muscle this size covering so much of the posterolateral rib cage will have an influence on diaphragmatic function. Any movement of the humerus will have an effect clear into the thoracolumbar fascia and further down the kinetic chain. Baby or satellite MtPs, consider; pectoralis major, teres major, subscapularis, triceps brachii, scalenes, upper rectus abdominis, iliocostalis, serratus anterior, serratus posterior superior and inferior, lower trapezius, and rhomboids.

Trigger point comment
LD generates pain in the mid-thoracic area including posterolateral abdominal pain. Pain of an aching nature in the inferior angle of the scapula and the posterior shoulder. Referred pain travels down the medial aspect of the humerus into the forearm, hand, and fingers.

Nerve
Thoracodorsal nerve, C6–C8.

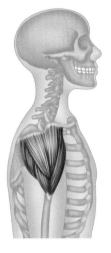

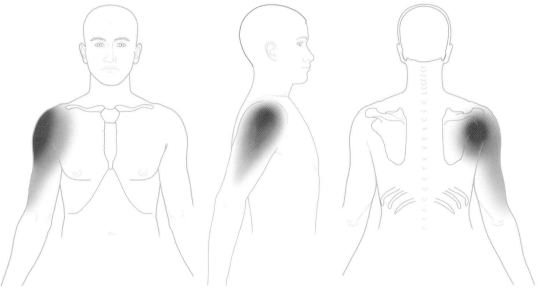

Muscle name
Deltoideus.

Greek, *delta*, fourth letter of Greek alphabet (shaped like a triangle).

Origin
Lateral third of clavicle, acromion, spine of scapula to deltoid tubercle.

Insertion
Middle of lateral surface of humerus (deltoid tuberosity).

Action
Abducts arm, anterior fibres flex and medially rotate, posterior fibres extend and laterally rotate.

Kinetic chain comment
This muscle, along with supraspinatus and associated rotator cuff muscles, will regularly develop trigger points due to reduced core efficiency. Failure to translate forces from the lower body to the shoulder will result in arthrokinematic stress and formation of active trigger points. Restoration of core neuromuscular efficiency will provide the foundation of trigger point therapy utilizing NMT and medical exercise.

Trigger point comment
Pain is felt as a dull ache for the most part with increased pain on contraction of the muscle or when attempts are made to move the arm. Pain is most often mistaken for bursitis or rotator cuff injury. It is worthwhile checking muscles that refer pain into the deltoid (SITS, pectorals, and scalenes) as the true source of deltoid pain. The deltoid trigger points are more often than not, *satellite trigger points*.

Nerve
Axillary nerve, C5, 6 (from posterior cord of the brachial plexus).

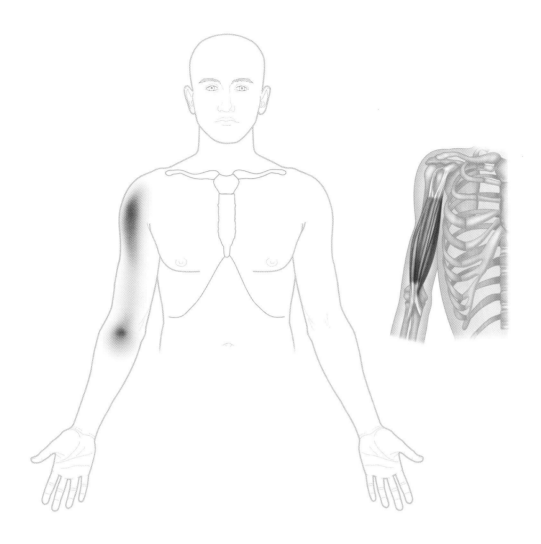

Muscle name
Biceps brachii.

Latin, *biceps*, two-headed muscle; *brachii*, of the arm.

Origin
Short head: A flat tendon shared with the coracobrachialis from the apex of the coracoid process of the scapula.
Long head: Arising from the supraglenoid tubercle of the scapula and the adjacent glenoid labrum of the glenohumeral joint.

Insertion
Posterior part of the tuberosity of radius, and the aponeurosis of the biceps brachii.

Action
With the origin fixed, flexion will occur at the elbow, initiating supination of the forearm. With the insertion fixed, the humerus is moved towards the forearm. The biceps brachii is also an important flexor of the shoulder joint through the action of the long head and an important shoulder stabilizer.

Kinetic chain comment
The biceps brachii decelerates extension and pronation at the elbow and extension at the shoulder joint. An important junction providing a fascial relationship between the thumb and the rib cage. Biceps brachii plays a vital role in shoulder stability under dynamic conditions, and can contract with the triceps brachii to stabilize the elbow.

Trigger point comment
Trigger points typically evolve in the centre of the gastor and refer pain up toward the anterior deltoid and down toward the pronator teres just distal to the elbow joint. NMT hypothesis includes weak core stability with poor neuromuscular efficiency culminating in compensatory trigger point formation to provide additional tension.

Nerve
Musculocutaneous nerve, C5, 6.

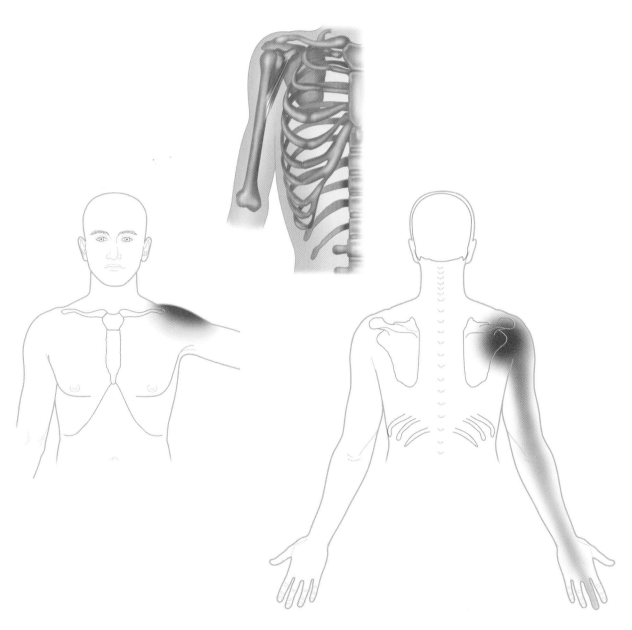

Muscle name
Coracobrachialis.

Greek, *coracoid*, raven's beak; **Latin**, *brachial*, relating to the arm.

Origin
Coracoid process of scapula with biceps brachii.

Insertion
Upper half medial border of humerus.

Action
Flexes and weakly adducts arm.

Kinetic chain comment
This muscle links the thoracic cage and the scapula with the arm. It does this as it shares the tendinous root onto the coracoid process with the pectoralis minor. Raising the arm out into abduction with the hand at the level of the ear demonstrates the continuity from the pectoralis minor through the coracobrachialis into the periosteum of the upper limb and travelling on through the brachioradialis all the way to the radial styloid.

Trigger point comment
Pain and/or numbness can be felt as far away as the posterior surface of the hand and into the middle finger. Pain can be referred to the posterior forearm, triceps brachii, and the anterior deltoid.

Nerve
Musculocutaneous nerve, C5–C7 (from lateral cord).

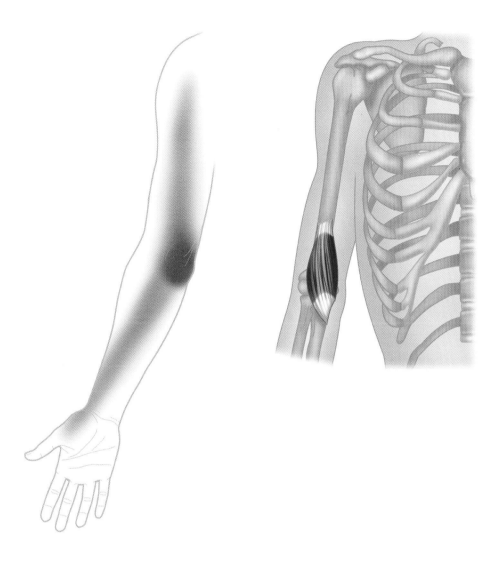

Muscle name
Brachialis.

Latin, *brachial*, relating to the arm.

Origin
Anterior lower half of humerus and medial and lateral intermuscular septa.

Insertion
Coronoid process and tuberosity of ulna.

Action
Flexes elbow.

Kinetic chain comment
An important link muscle in the chain, linking the thorax with the upper limb. This muscle has the ability to trap the radial nerve resulting in numbness or other nerve-related sensations including dysesthesia of the thumb. Of course such symptoms could also be caused by trigger points.

Trigger point comment
Pain spreads to the base of the thumb, anterior deltoid and just below the elbow joint line. Patients often complain of tingling or numbness in the thumb and hand. These problems can be misdiagnosed as carpal tunnel syndrome.

Nerve
Musculocutaneous nerve, C5, 6 (from lateral cord). Also small supply from radial nerve, C7.

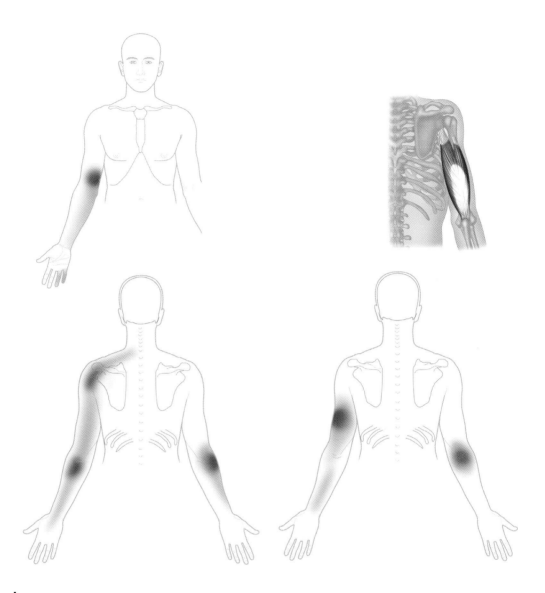

Muscle name
Triceps brachii.

Latin, *triceps*, three-headed muscle; *brachii*, of the arm.

Origin
Long head: Infraglenoid tubercle of scapula.
Lateral head: Upper half posterior humerus (linear origin).
Medial head: Lies deep on lower half posterior humerus inferomedial to spiral groove and both intermuscular septa.

Insertion
Posterior part of upper surface of olecranon process of ulna and posterior capsule.

Action
Extends elbow. The long head stabilizes the shoulder joint. The medial head retracts the capsule of the elbow joint on extension.

Kinetic chain comment
Triceps brachii assists deceleration of flexion at the glenohumeral joint and the elbow joint along with its 'little helper', *anconeus*. The radial nerve can be irritated by contracture or spasm of the lateral aspect of this muscle.

Trigger point comment
Pain can be felt in the neck and upper trapezius. Other symptoms make it easy to misdiagnose pain felt in the elbow and triceps brachii as tennis or golfer's elbow. Trigger points in this muscle make it difficult to extend the arm at the elbow. Patients complain that they cannot rest their elbow on any surface due to the level of sensitivity and pain.

Nerve
Radial nerve, C6–C8, T1.

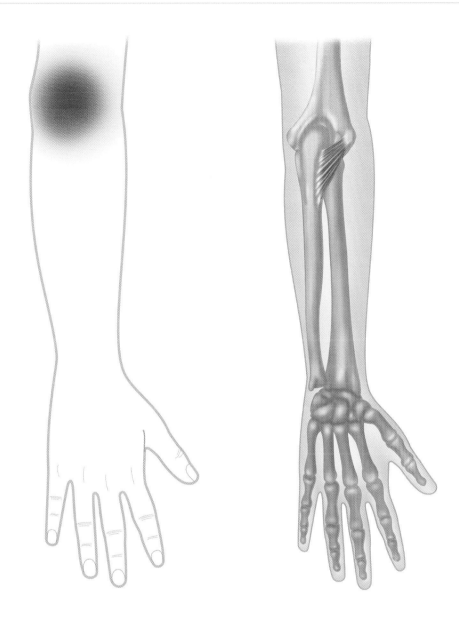

Muscle name
Anconeus.

Greek, elbow.

Origin
Smooth surface at lower extremity of posterior aspect of lateral epicondyle of the humerus.

Insertion
Lateral side of olecranon.

Action
Weak extensor of elbow and abducts the ulna in pronation.

Kinetic chain comment
Anconeus decelerates elbow flexion and supination. These trigger points typically evolve due to active trigger points in more superior and medial muscles of the neck and shoulder. Trigger points can evolve here due to gripping too tightly (e.g. a golf club, tennis racket, or writing pen) but reduced core strength must be considered as a causative factor.

Trigger point comment
Pain from trigger points in this muscle are mistaken for lateral epicondylitis or tennis elbow. Difficulty and pain will be experienced trying to flex the elbow joint and in supination of the forearm.

Nerve
Radial nerve, C7, 8.

Muscles of the Shoulder, Arm, and Hand

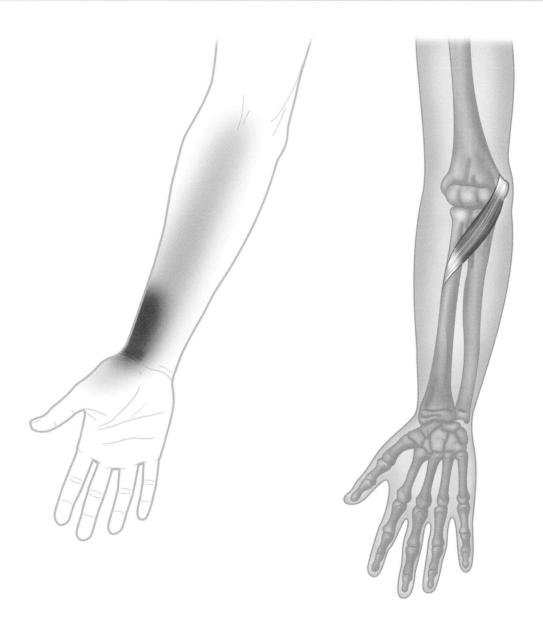

Muscle name
Pronator teres.

Latin, *pronate*, bent forward; *teres*, rounded, finely shaped.

Origin
Medial epicondyle of the humerus and coronoid process of the ulna.

Insertion
Middle of lateral surface of the radius.

Action
Pronates and flexes forearm at the elbow.

Kinetic chain comment
Decelerates supination and extension of the forearm at the elbow.

Trigger point comment
Pain on the ulnar side of the forearm and at the base of the thumb. Difficulty turning the palm into supination with extension without pain and stiffness. Patient's have difficulty cupping the hand.

Nerve
Median nerve, C6, 7.

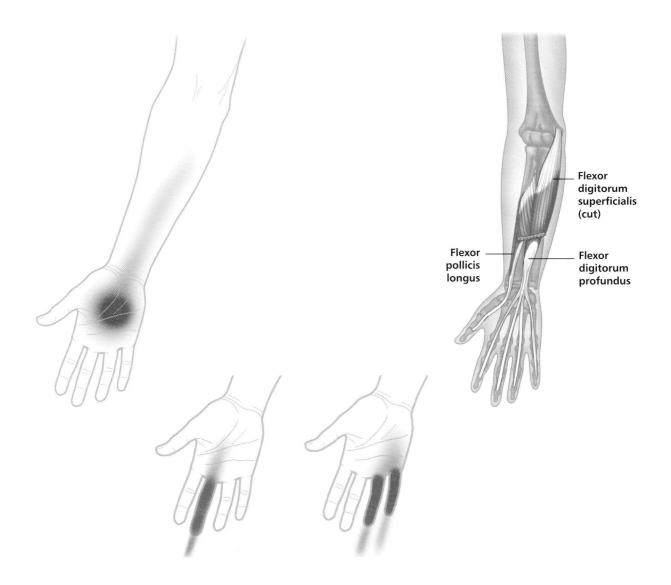

Flexor digitorum superficialis (cut)

Flexor pollicis longus

Flexor digitorum profundus

Muscle name
Forearm flexors.

Latin, *flex*, to bend.

Origin
Medial epicondyle of the humerus.

Insertion
Digits of the hand; the carpals, metacarpals, and thumb.

Action
Flexion of the wrist and fingers.

Kinetic chain comment
A common theme in this textbook is the notion that the upper limb relies on forces to be translated from the lower limbs through the core, so that the arms can carry out some function. Lack of core stability will lead to these muscles developing extra stiffness in an effort to provide the forces required when communication has been broken within the kinetic chain. Habitual tasks will determine which muscles shorten and which become inhibited. Typically the forearm flexors will shorten while the extensors become inhibited. Treatment of the flexors first can often yield best results followed by medical exercise to build extensor endurance and tone.

Trigger point comment
As there are numerous muscles in this area, variations of pain patterns will be influenced by specific muscles. In general, these trigger points refer pain into the anterior part of the hand and lateral three fingers. Spray and stretch technique is particularly good in the treatment of these muscles and restoration of homeostasis.

Nerve
Radial and ulnar nerves.

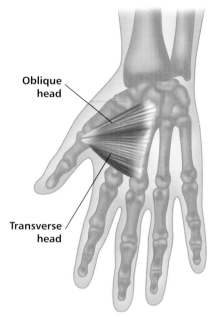

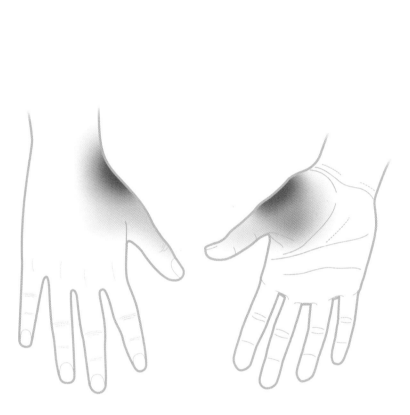

Muscle name
Adductor pollicis.

Latin, *adduct*, toward; *pollicis*, of the thumb.

Origin
Flexor retinaculum and tubercles of scaphoid and trapezium.

Insertion
Lateral side of base of proximal phalanx of thumb.

Action
Abducts thumb and helps oppose it.

Kinetic chain comment
This muscle decelerates abduction of the thumb and extension of the metacarpophalangeal joint of the thumb.

Trigger point comment
Aching pain is felt on the outside of the thumb and hand at the base of the thumb which has a tendency to lock. Patients find it difficult to control movement of the thumb and their handwriting can become illegible, with difficulty holding a pen. A frustration builds when they have difficulty closing buttons or performing actions that require fine muscle control.

Trigger point pain can be felt in the thumb web space and thenar eminence. It is worth pointing out at this stage to remember what other muscles refer pain into these areas. Scalenes, brachialis, supinator, extensor carpi radialis longus, and brachioradialis. Remember to check these muscles first (in the order of most medial and superior).

Nerve
Deep ulnar nerve, C8, T1.

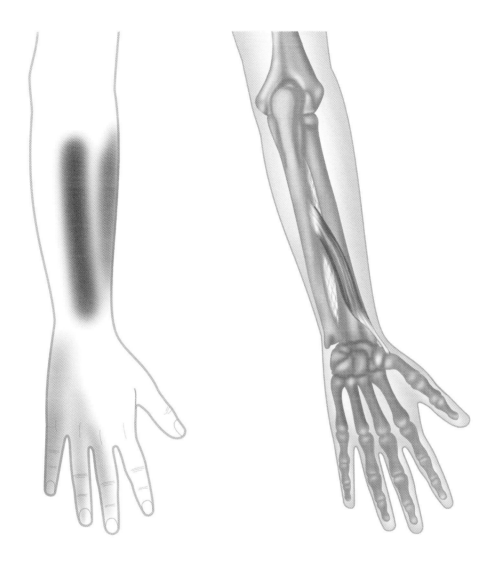

Muscle name
Abductor pollicis longus.

Latin, *abduct*, away from; *pollicis*, of the thumb; *longus*, long.

Origin
Posterior surfaces of ulna, radius, and interosseous membrane.

Insertion
The base of the first metacarpal.

Action
Abducts and extends the thumb at the carpometacarpal joint.

Kinetic chain comment
This muscle decelerates adduction of the thumb.

Trigger point comment
Abductor pollicis longus is one of a number of muscles that can generate stiffness in the hand and fingers, often mistaken for arthritis. Patients report waking from their sleep due to cramping. Due to inhibitory influences, the fingers and forearm lose local endurance, and fatigue sets in early on. Skilled control of the thumb reduces.

Referred pain patterns of the abductor pollicis longus resemble the C6, 7, and 8 dermatomes, the superficial radial sensory nerve distribution, and are very similar to the area of pain experienced in De Quervain's tenosynovitis. Identification of the abductor pollicis longus trigger points should be considered in pain of the radial aspect of the wrist and thumb, especially when other neurological abnormalities or inflammatory conditions have been ruled out.

Nerve
Posterior interosseous nerve, C6–C8.

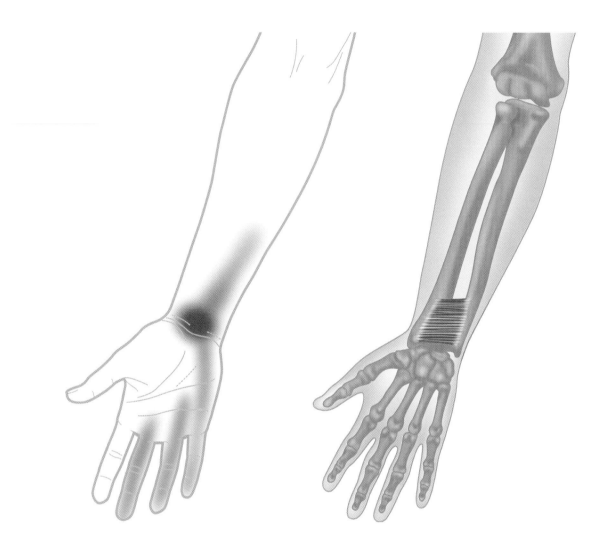

Muscle name
Pronator quadratus (PQ).

Latin, *pronate*, bent forward; *quadratus*, squared.

Origin
Distal quarter of shaft of ulna.

Insertion
Distal shaft of radius.

Action
Pronates forearm; deep fibres bind radius and ulna together.

Trigger point comment
Two main pain patterns are observed. The most common pattern involves pain spreading both distally and proximally along the medial aspect of the forearm. In some cases, the pain area extends to the medial epicondyle proximally and the fifth digit distally. The second main pattern is pain spreading distally to the third and/or fourth finger. The pain patterns originating from the PQ resemble the C8–T1 dermatomes, and ulnar and median nerve sensory distributions. Therefore, myofascial pain of the PQ should be considered as a possible cause of pain in the medial forearm and hand, especially when other neurological abnormalities have been ruled out.

Kinetic chain comment
Failure to stabilize the relationship between the radius and ulna leads to complications along the upper limb fascial sleeve resulting in shoulder joint and shoulder girdle/neck problems. Attempts to strengthen the forearm with increases in weight training or similar will result in compounding the patient's problems. PQ must have its myofascial trigger points dealt with before an appropriate course of physical activity is introduced with an emphasis on endurance.

Nerve
Anterior interosseous from median nerve, C7, 8, T1.

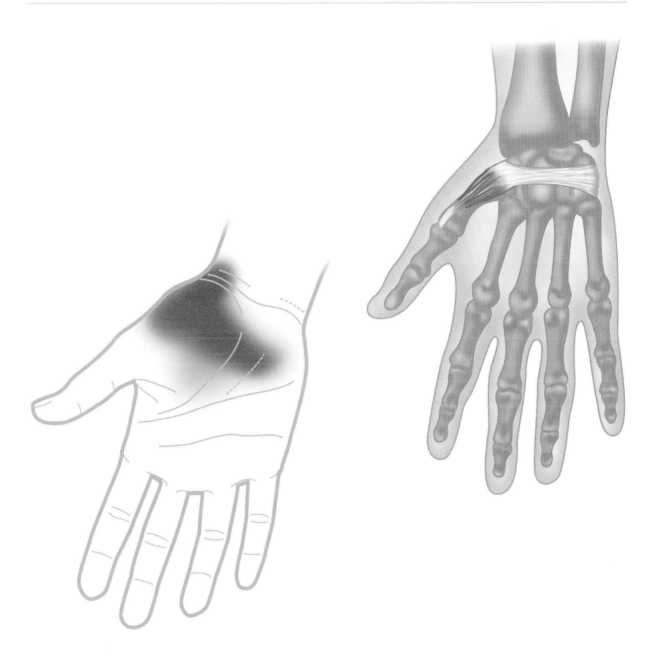

Muscle name

Abductor pollicis brevis.

Latin, *abduct*, away from; *pollicis*, of the thumb; *brevis*, short.

Origin

Flexor retinaculum, transverse carpal ligament, and tubercles of the scaphoid and trapezium.

Insertion

Attaching to the lateral side of base of proximal phalanx of the thumb.

Action

Abducts the thumb and helps to oppose it.

Kinetic chain comment

Decelerates adduction of the thumb.

Trigger point comment

Patient's will report a loss of grip strength. Pain and sensations are experienced in the palmar aspect of the thumb and wrist (radial side).

Nerve

Recurrent branch of median nerve, C7, 8, and T1.

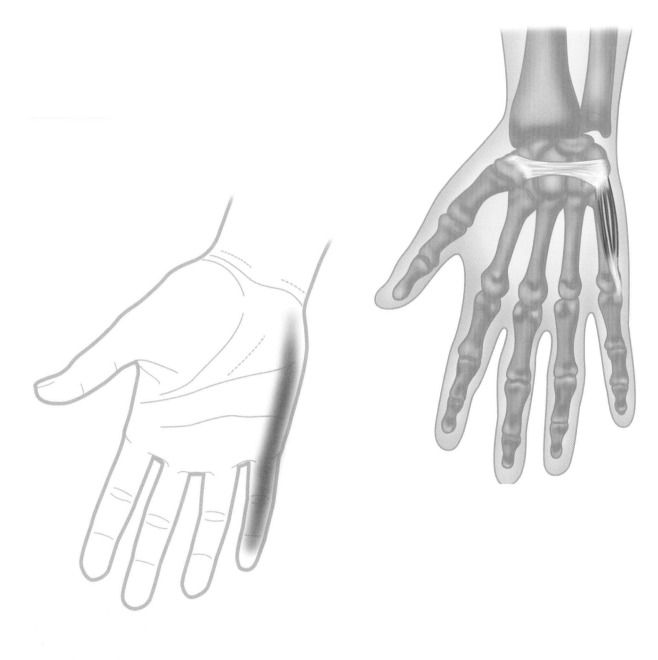

Muscle name
Abductor digiti minimi.

Latin, *abductor*, away from; *digit*, finger; *minimi*, shortest.

Origin
Pisiform bone and the tendon of the flexor carpi ulnaris.

Insertion
Medial side of base of proximal phalanx of the little finger.

Action
Abducts the fifth (little) finger.

Kinetic chain comment
Decelerates adduction of the fifth finger.

Trigger point comment
As the name of the muscle would suggest, pain and stiffness is felt in the little finger and is often described as being an arthritic type pain.

Nerve
Deep branch of ulnar nerve, C8 and T1.

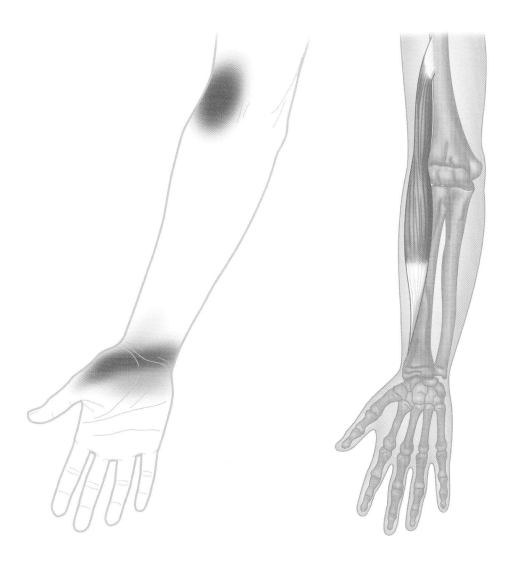

Muscle name
Brachioradialis.

Latin, *brachial*, relating to the arm; *radius*, staff, spoke of wheel.

Origin
Proximal two-thirds of lateral supracondyle ridge of humerus and lateral intermuscular septal fascia.

Insertion
Lateral surface of distal end of radial styloid process.

Action
Flexes the elbow joint and assists in pronation and supination of the forearm.

Kinetic chain comment
This is an important muscle in joining the forearm and anatomical arm decelerating extension of the forearm at the elbow. This is a classical example of a 'shunt muscle', preventing, as it does, separation of the elbow joint during rapid movements. Baby or satellite myofascial trigger points should include the supinator, extensor carpi radialis longus, triceps brachii, and extensor digitorum.

Trigger point comment
Known as the 'politician's trigger point' as a result of shaking hands so often with so many voters. Pain is referred to the wrist and the base of the thumb in the web space. Also pain is felt at the lateral epicondyle. A full examination of all the associated muscles in the kinetic chain must be carried out as it is difficult to know for sure which muscle is the major or true source of pain.

Nerve
Radial nerve, C5, 6.

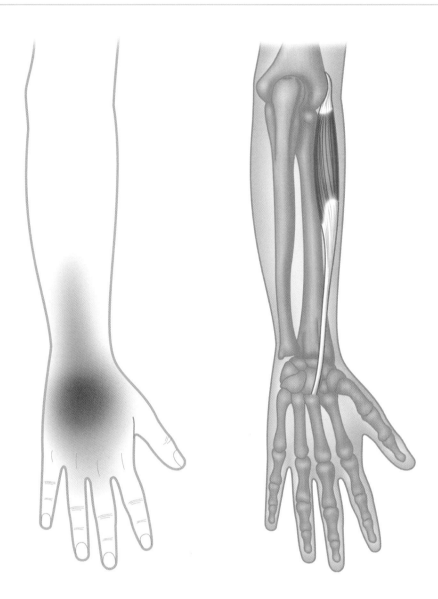

Muscle name
Extensor carpi radialis brevis.

Latin, *extensor*, to extend; *carpi*, of the wrist; *radius*, staff, spoke of wheel; *brevis*, short.

Origin
Lateral epicondyle of humerus.

Insertion
Posterior base of the third metacarpal bone.

Action
Extends the wrist and hand and abducts the hand.

Kinetic chain comment
Decelerates flexion of the wrist and hand and adduction of the hand. Baby or satellite myofascial trigger points to consider include supinator, brachioradialis, and triceps brachii.

Trigger point comment
Wrist and hand pain are a common feature of these myofascial trigger points with noted stiffness in the morning and increased pain on bending the fingers. Difficulty sustaining a grip on handles or golf clubs is reported due to a noticeable increase in weakness of the associated muscles. Changes in sensations include tingling, pins and needles, and numbness. Often mistaken for tendonitis.

Nerve
Radial nerve, C5–C8.

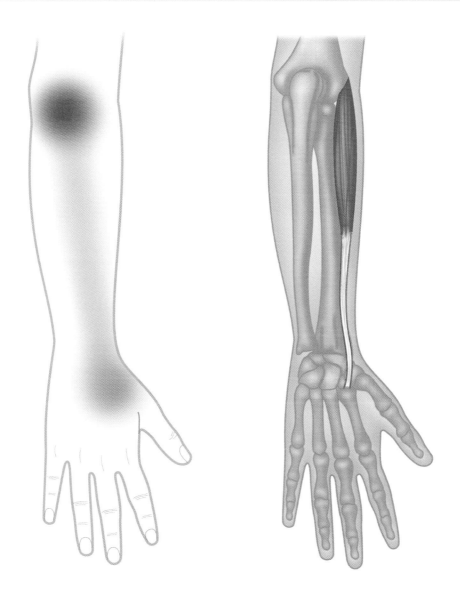

Muscle name
Extensor carpi radialis longus.

Latin, *extensor*, to extend; *carpi*, of the wrist; *radius*, staff, spoke of wheel; *longus*, long.

Origin
Lateral supracondyle ridge (inferior third) of humerus and lateral intermuscular septum.

Insertion
Dorsal base of the second metacarpal.

Action
Extends and abducts the hand at the wrist joint.

Trigger point comment
Myofascial trigger points (MtPs) in this muscle lead to severe, unrelenting lateral epicondylitis. Failure to treat these MtPs will result in the tennis elbow constantly returning – a great example of treating the symptom and not the cause. My patients complain of an unrelenting burning sensation with a focus on the elbow and referred pain into the wrist and the fleshy part between the thumb and the fourth digit known as the *anatomical snuffbox*.

Nerve
Radial nerve, C5–C8.

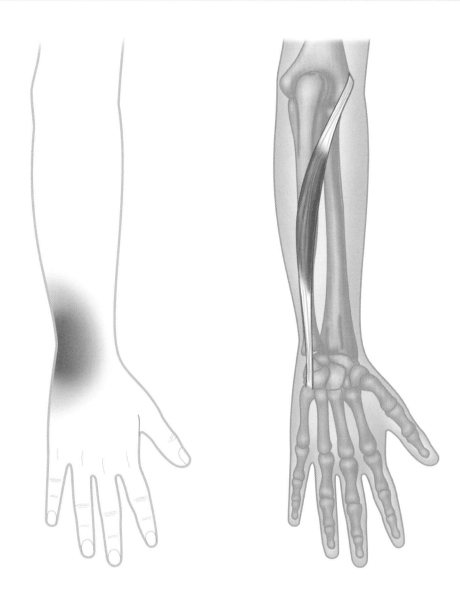

Muscle name
Extensor carpi ulnaris.

Latin, *extensor*, to extend; *carpi*, of the wrist; *ulnaris*, of the elbow.

Origin
Lateral epicondyle of humerus and posterior border of ulna.

Insertion
Base of the fifth metacarpal.

Action
Extends and adducts the hand at the wrist joint.

Kinetic chain comment
Decelerates flexion and abduction of the hand at the wrist. Baby or satellite myofascial trigger points for consideration should include extensor digitorum and brachioradialis.

Trigger point comment
Pain is referred to the ulnar aspect of the posterior wrist often mistaken for a wrist sprain. Sensations include burning or numbness.

Nerve
Posterior interosseous (radial) nerve, C6–C8.

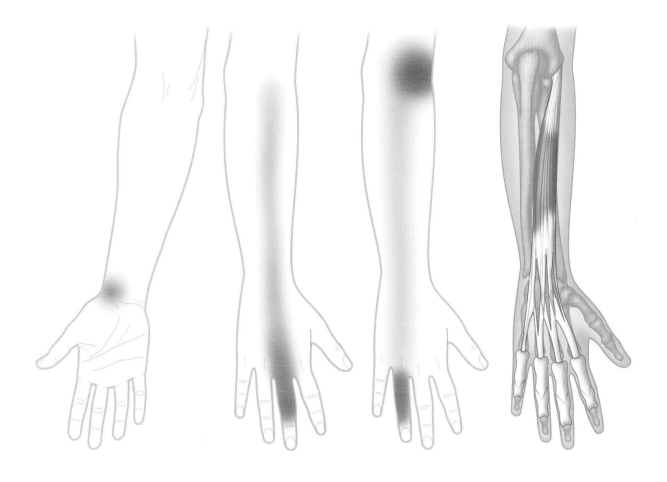

Muscle name
Extensor digitorum.

Latin, *extensor*, to extend; *digit*, finger.

Origin
Lateral epicondyle of humerus.

Insertion
Extensor expansions of medial four digits.

Action
Extends medial four digits (not the thumb) at the metacarpophalangeal joints. Extends the hand at the wrist joint.

Kinetic chain comment
A decelerator of the fingers, hands, and wrist through flexion. A good assessment is the finger flexion test where you ask the patient to touch the pads of their fingers (i.e. fingertips) to the palmar pads while the metacarpophalangeal joints are held straight. All fingers should touch the palmar surface. Failure to do so would demonstrate shortness in the muscle/s, most likely requiring treatment. Responsible for baby or satellite MtPs in supinator, brachioradialis, extensor carpi radialis longus, and extensor carpi ulnaris.

Trigger point comment
Pain, stiffness, cramping and weakness are the common sensations reported. Pain down the forearm to the posterior part of the hand into the middle finger. Pain can be confused with lateral epicondylitis, C7 radiculopathy and De Quervain's stenosing tenosynovitis. All the associated muscles such as extensor indicis, digitorum, and digiti minimi must be considered and appropriately treated when pain in the fingers is the chief complaint.

Nerve
Posterior interosseous nerve, C6–C8.

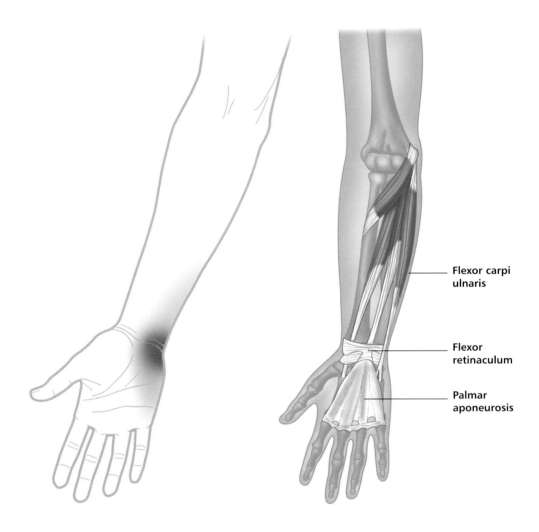

Flexor carpi
ulnaris

Flexor
retinaculum

Palmar
aponeurosis

Muscle name
Flexor carpi ulnaris (FCU).

Latin, *flex*, to bend; *carpi*, of the wrist; *ulnaris*, of the elbow/arm.

Origin
The humeral head of FCU attaches to the medial epicondyle of the humerus, while the ulnar head attaches from the olecranon process and the proximal posterior ulna.

Insertion
Base of the second metacarpal/pisiform bone and a portion of the third metacarpal/hamate and fifth metacarpal bones.

Action
Both flexes and abducts the wrist and provides weak pronation of the forearm and elbow flexion.

Kinetic chain comment
Decelerates flexion and abduction of the wrist and hand and extension of the forearm at the elbow.

Trigger point comment
Numbness and burning sensations can be experienced in the third, fourth, and fifth fingers. Pain is reported on the medial aspect (little finger side) of the wrist as a sharp pain that can spread across the wrist joint giving rise to misdiagnosis of carpal tunnel or wrist sprains, medial epicondylitis, ulnar neuropathy, carpal tunnel syndrome, Charcot's arthropathy, rheumatoid arthritis, osteoarthritis, C5 radiculopathy, peripheral neuropathy, Dupuytren's contracture, diabetic neuropathy, polyneuropathy, systemic lupus erythematosus, complex regional pain syndrome (reflex sympathetic dystrophy), systemic infections, or inflammation. Of course these must be ruled out by a primary medical practitioner and so if in doubt, refer.

Nerve
Ulnar nerve, C7, 8, T1.

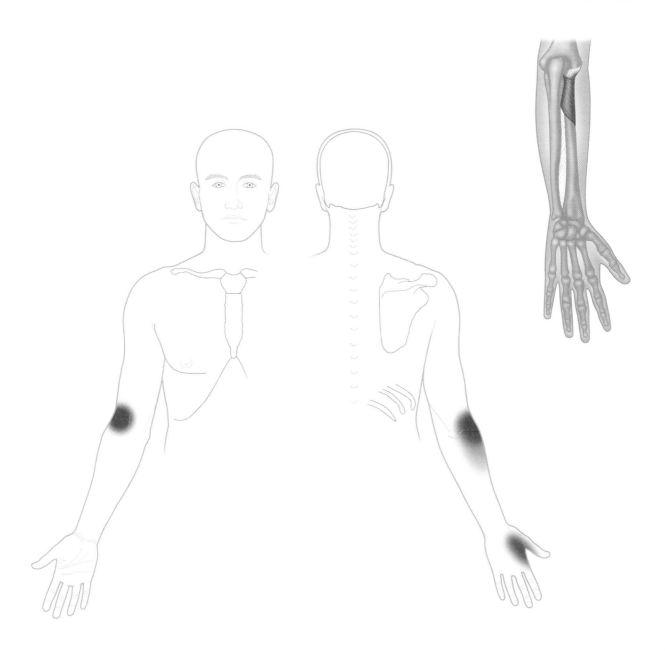

Muscle name
Supinator.

Latin, *supinus*, lying on the back.

Origin
Lateral epicondyle of humerus, radial collateral ligament of elbow joint, and the annular ligament of the radius including the superior crest of the ulna.

Insertion
Lateral upper one third of the radius.

Action
Supinates the forearm and the hand.

Kinetic chain comment
The supinator is associated with deceleration of the elbow during extension. When the forearm is held between supination and pronation, the supinator will decelerate elbow extension.

Trigger point comment
A lateral elbow pain generator. This muscle sneaks pain down into the web of the thumb on the dorsal side. Changes in sensations include, but are not limited to, numbness and weakness in the hand (this may be due to compression of the deep branch of the radial nerve-posterior interosseous nerve), and fingers.

Nerve
Deep branch of radial nerve, C5–C7.

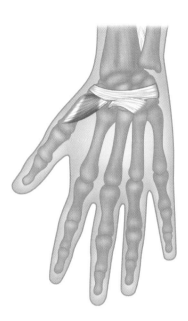

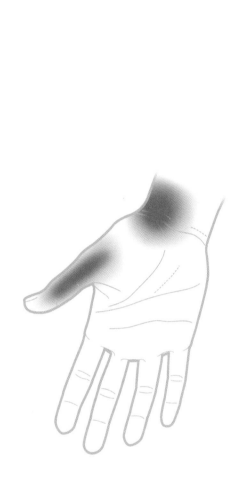

Muscle name
Opponens pollicis.

Latin, *opponens*, opposing; *pollicis*, of the thumb.

Origin
Flexor retinaculum and tubercles of scaphoid and trapezium.

Insertion
Lateral side of the first metacarpal.

Action
Moves the first metacarpal laterally opposing the thumb toward the centre of the palm and rotating it medially.

Kinetic chain comment
Decelerates adduction and extension with return from opposition. May lead to what Travell and Simons say patients refer to as *clumsy thumb*.

Trigger point comment
Pain refers to the palmar surface of both the thumb and wrist. It has been reported that many patients can identify a specific point on the radial side of the palmar aspect of the wrist as being the source of the pain. It has been mistaken for C6 or C7 radiculopathy, carpal tunnel syndrome, De Quervain's stenosing tenosynovitis, carpometacarpal dysfunction, osteoarthritis, articular dysfunction, paronychia (ingrown thumbnail), bone cancer, bone fracture, strain/sprain, rheumatoid arthritis, Dupuytren's contracture, ganglion cyst, mixed connective tissue disease, Raynaud's phenomenon, frostbite, diabetic neuropathy, systemic infections or inflammation, nutritional inadequacy, metabolic imbalance, toxicity and side-effects of medications.

Nerve
Median nerve, C6–C8, T1.

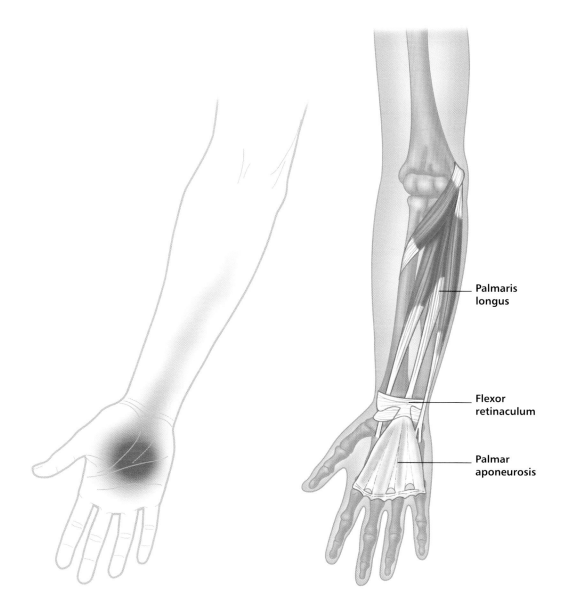

Palmaris longus

Flexor retinaculum

Palmar aponeurosis

Muscle name
Palmaris longus.

Latin, *palmaris*, palma, palm; *longus*, long.

Origin
Medial epicondyle of humerus.

Insertion
Distal half of flexor retinaculum and palmar aponeurosis and transverse carpal ligament.

Action
Flexes hand at the wrist, stiffens the aponeurosis of the palm and assists in pronation and flexion of the forearm.

Kinetic chain comment
Decelerates extension of the hand at the wrist whilst decelerating supination of the hand against gravity and extension of the forearm at the elbow.

Trigger point comment
A focal point of pain from this muscle is experienced as a needle-like sensation rather than the deep aching pain of MtPs in many other muscles. Pain can extend to the base of the thumb and distal crease of the palm. A residue of this pain can travel to the distal volar forearm.

Nerve
Median nerve, C7, 8, T1.

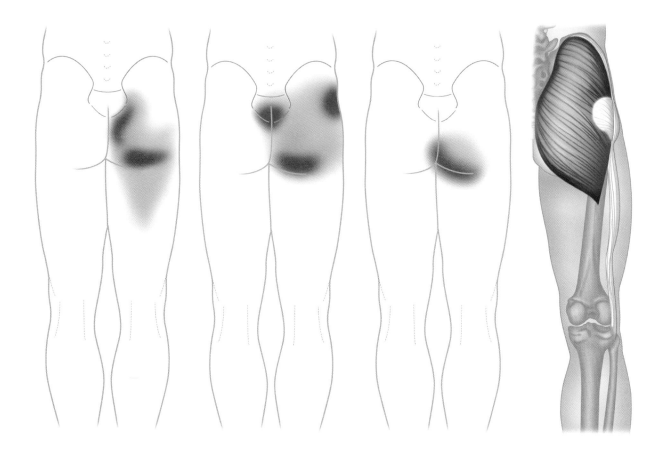

Muscle name
Gluteus maximus.

Greek, *gloutos*, buttock; *maximus*, biggest.

Origin
Gluteal surface of the ilium behind the posterior gluteal line, posterior border of the ilium, aponeurosis of erector spinae, sacrotuberous ligament and gluteal aponeurosis.

Insertion
Iliotibial band of fascia lata and gluteal tuberosity of the femur by means of a broad aponeurosis.

Action
Laterally rotates and extends the hip joint while assists in adduction at the hip joint. Eccentrically, gluteus maximus contracts to decelerate hip flexion, adduction, and internal rotation.

Kinetic chain comment
Gluteus maximus has a significant role to play in stabilizing both the sacroiliac joint and the knee joint. It does so by means of superior fibres, which attach to the aponeurosis of the sacrotuberous ligament and inferior fibres attaching anteriorly to the iliotibial band providing tension down to the knee. Weak gluteals have wide reaching implications up and down the kinetic chain.

Trigger point comment
It is hypothesised that gluteal trigger points could be as a result of inhibition to the gluteals caused by spasm in the psoas muscles, gluteus medius and minimus. The formation of these trigger points providing much needed tension for sacroiliac support. Pain is often felt in the lower back and mimics bursitis of the hip with pain experienced at the site of the coccygeal bone and gluteal crease. Weakness in gluteus maximus can be resolved by finding which trigger points are referring the inhibition to it. Gluteus maximus requires specific retraining following appropriate treatment. It commonly causes abnormal gait that aggravates all sorts of other problems, including the knee.

Nerve
Inferior gluteal nerve, L5, S1, 2.

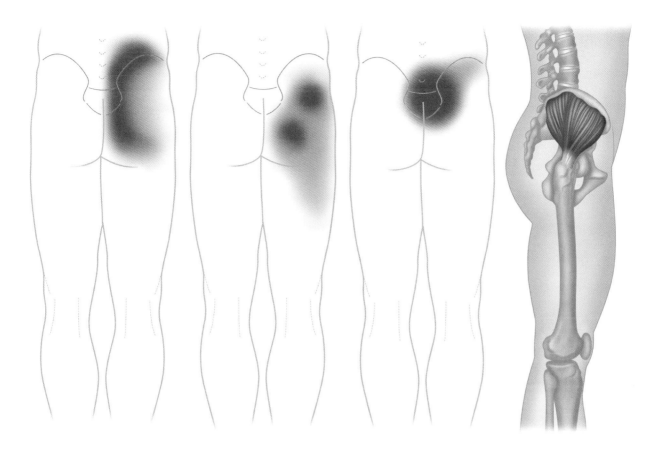

Muscle name
Gluteus medius.

Greek, *gloutos*, buttock; *medius*, middle.

Origin
Outer surface of ilium between posterior and middle gluteal lines.

Insertion
Posterolateral surface of greater trochanter of femur.

Action
Abducts and both externally/internally rotates the hip. Tilts pelvis on walking.

Kinetic chain comment
This muscle is a crucial muscle in offering stability to the lateral line. Weak gluteus medius leads to low back pain for runners and creates undue knee stress. This pain is often mistaken for discogenic problems and sacroiliac dysfunction. Standing one leg test (Stork test) will often result in the patient being unable to stabilize the iliofemoral relationship on the frontal plane as the gluteus medius is required to eccentrically contract or decelerate the movement. This can be evident as an exaggerated lateral hip sway during walking due to over-pronation of the foot, dropped arch, rotation of the second toe (Morton's foot) and medial rotation of the tibia/femur. Baby or satellite myofascial trigger points include quadratus lumborum, piriformis, gluteus minimus, gluteus maximus, and tensor fasciae latae.

Trigger point comment
Low back pain is felt above and below the belt line. Pain in the hips makes it difficult to sleep in comfort and leads to disturbed sleep patterns. This muscle is a major generator of low back and hip pain, as well as complaints of a burning sensation along the PSIS and sacroiliac joint. Often mistaken for lumbago type pain and discomfort (such as tenderness) into the buttocks and superior thigh.

Nerve
Superior gluteal nerve, L4, 5, S1.

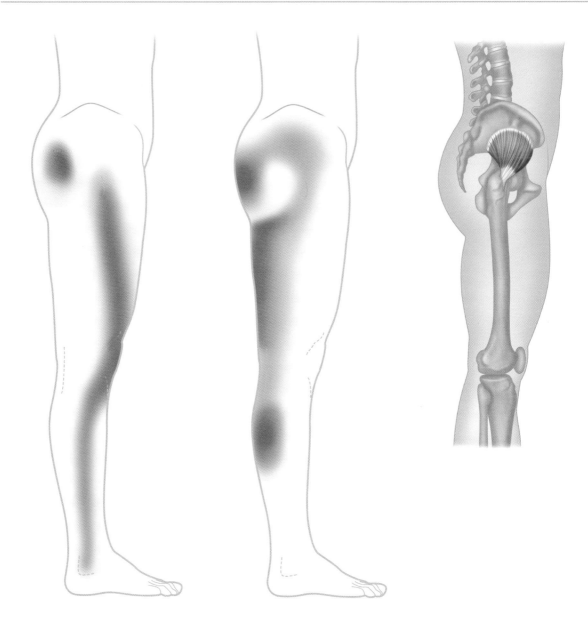

Muscle name
Gluteus minimus.

Greek, *gloutos*, buttock; *minimus*, smallest.

Origin
Outer surface of ilium between middle and inferior gluteal lines.

Insertion
Anterior surface of greater trochanter of femur.

Action
Abducts and medially rotates hip. Assists in tilting the pelvis when walking.

Trigger point comment
Pain is experienced in the posterior and/or lateral thigh as well as deep in the buttocks. Numbness can be another symptom and pain can refer as far as the lateral ankle. Such pain and discomfort can be mistaken for sciatic pain.

Kinetic chain comment
Gluteus minimus acts to decelerate external rotation and adduction of the femur in the hip joint.

Nerve
Superior gluteal nerve, L4, 5, S1.

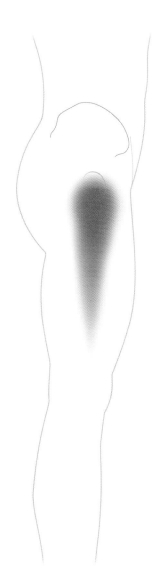

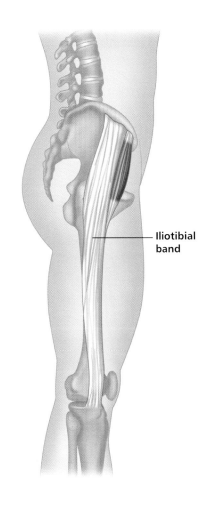

Iliotibial band

Muscle name
Tensor fasciae latae.

Latin, *tensor*, stretcher, puller; *fascia(e)*, band(s); *latae*, broad.

Origin
Anterior superior iliac spine, outer lip of anterior iliac crest and fascia lata.

Insertion
Iliotibial band.

Action
Assists to stabilize and steady the hip and knee joints by putting tension on the iliotibial band of fascia.

Kinetic chain comment
Tensor fasciae latae is a vitally important structure in providing stability through the knee and pelvis. This muscle is a junction for several chains including the spiral and lateral chains. Anteromedial fibres are responsible for flexion of the thigh while posterolateral fibres provide stability for the knee. Tensor fasciae latae assists muscles including gluteus medius, minimus, rectus femoris, iliopsoas, pectineus, and sartorius.

Trigger point comment
Pain is felt at the level of the greater trochanter in the hip joint. Walking and running activities make the pain more intense. Pain can refer midway down the lateral thigh and can cause additional knee pain.

Nerve
Superior gluteal nerve, L4, 5, S1.

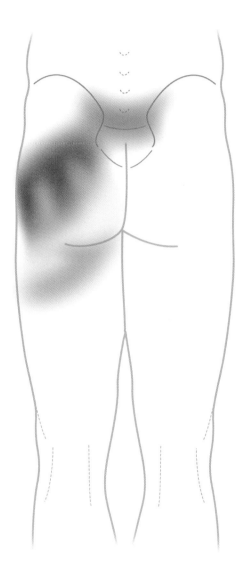

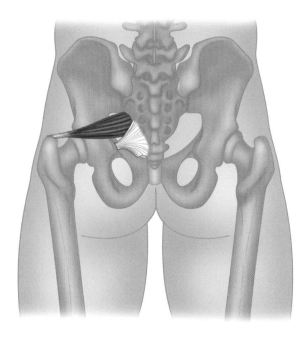

Muscle name
Piriformis.

Latin, *pirum*, a pear; *piriform*, pear-shaped.

Origin
Second, third, and fourth costotransverse bars of anterior sacrum, a small number of fibres arise from the superior border of the greater sciatic notch.

Insertion
Superior border of greater trochanter of the femur.

Action
Laterally rotates the hip and abducts the thigh when the hip is flexed.

Kinetic chain comment
Piriformis eccentrically contracts to decelerate internal rotation and hip adduction when the hip is flexed. Short piriformis can cause the sacrum to tilt giving the appearance of a short leg discrepancy and cause a rotation or twisting of the sacrum in the sacroiliac joint, setting up additional sacroiliac stress. This is a recipe for shoulder injury if not corrected in a timely fashion.

Trigger point comment
This pain is felt in the buttock, hip, and base of the spine, including the sacral base and at times into the upper hamstrings.

Nerve
Ventral rami of lumbar nerve, L5, and sacral nerves, S1, 2.

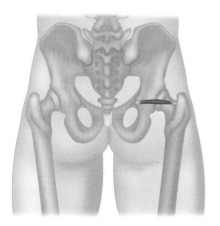

Gemellus superior

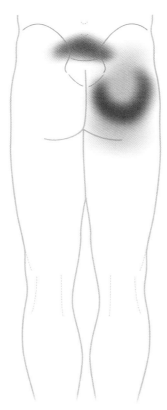

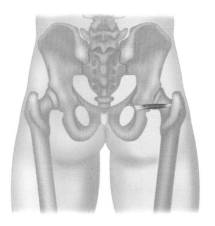

Gemellus inferior

Muscle name
Gemelli.

Latin, *gemellus*, a twin.

Origin
Upper border of ischial tuberosity (inferior), spine of ischium (superior).

Insertion
Middle part of medial aspect of greater trochanter of femur (inferior), middle part of medial aspect of greater trochanter of femur (superior).

Action
Laterally rotates and stabilizes the hip.

Kinetic chain comment
Any pain in the pelvic area will result in either an apprehension or a reluctance to movement. This often results in postural adaptations and changes in muscle synergies needed to carry out some function.

Trigger point comment
Interpelvic pain with difficulty sitting for even short periods of time. Intense and unrelenting pain can be referred into the base of the spine and also into the gluteal area. The gemelli and obturator muscles are difficult to treat with finger applications. Trigger points can be treated successfully with dry needling.

Nerve
Nerve to quadratus femoris, L4, 5, S1 (inferior). Nerve to obturator internus, L5, S1, 2 (superior).

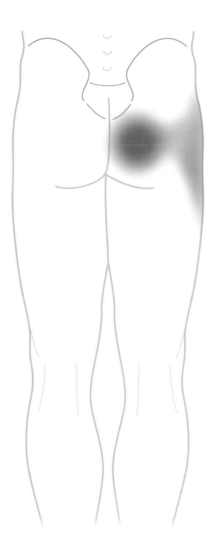

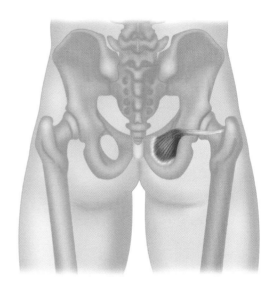

Muscle name
Obturator internus.

Latin, *obturator*, obstructor; *internus*, internal.

Origin
Pelvic surface of obturator membrane and bony margin of the obturator foramen.

Insertion
Anterior part of medial surface of greater trochanter of femur.

Action
Laterally rotates the extended thigh at the hip, stabilizes the hip, and produces horizontal extension. Abducts the flexed thigh.

Kinetic chain comment
Eccentric contraction decelerates internal rotation of the femur while pulling the head of the femur into the acetabulum to fix the femoral head during abduction. It eccentrically controls the head of the femur on returning from adduction.

Trigger point comment
Local pain is experienced deep within the pelvic basin and out as far as the anterior medial portion of the greater trochanter.

Nerve
Branch of the ventral rami of lumbar nerve, L5, and sacral nerves, S1, 2.

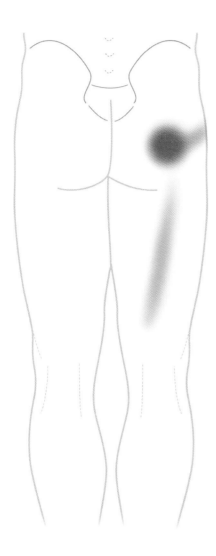

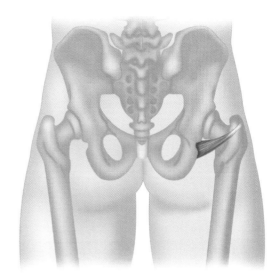

Muscle name
Obturator externus.

Latin, *obturator*, obstructor; *externus*, external.

Origin
Rami of pubis and ischium.

Insertion
Trochanteric fossa of femur.

Action
Laterally rotates and stabilizes the hip.

Kinetic chain comment
Eccentric contraction decelerates medial or internal rotation and abduction of the femur.

Trigger point comment
Local pain is experienced deep within the pelvic basin and out as far as the posterior portion of the greater trochanter. If resisted, medial rotation causes an increase in pain (sometimes the pain shoots down the medial aspect of the femur). This author has found that trigger points housed in the obturator externus may well be the culprit. This may be a worthwhile test to perform.

Nerve
Posterior division of the obturator nerve, L3, 4.

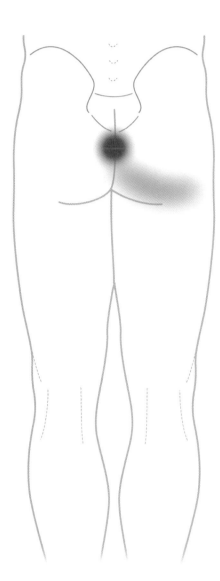

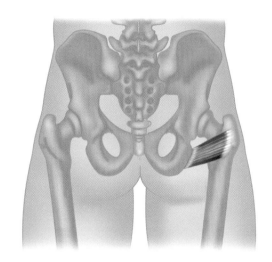

Muscle name
Quadratus femoris.

Latin, *quadratus*, squared; *femoris*, of the thigh.

Origin
Lateral border (superior aspect) of ischial tuberosity.

Insertion
Quadrate tubercle of femur and a vertical line below this to the level of lesser trochanter.

Action
Laterally rotates and stabilizes hip.

Kinetic chain comment
Eccentrically decelerates medial rotation of the femur at the hip.

Trigger point comment
Pain is felt locally in the posterior pubis and lower gluteal area. Difficulty in sleeping and walking downstairs are reported.

Nerve
Nerve to quadratus femoris, L4, 5, S1.

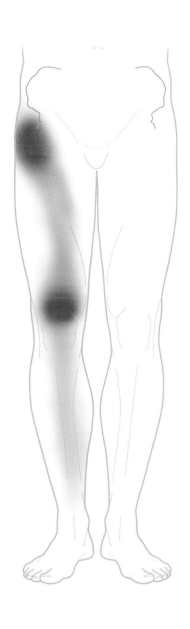

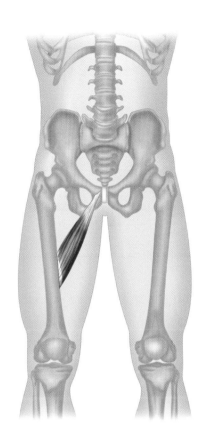

Muscle name

Adductor longus.

Latin, *adductor*, toward; *longus*, long.

Origin

Anterior of pubis in angle between the crest and symphysis.

Insertion

Middle third of the medial lip of the linea aspera.

Kinetic chain comment

Decelerates femoral external rotation and abduction of the thigh.

Trigger point comment

Patients presenting with groin pain should be considered for trigger points in their adductor longus. Pain can be felt deep in the hip joint, inner thigh and at the medial aspect of the knee. Sensations such as joint stiffness in the hip are reported, restricting ROM in all directions.

Nerve

Anterior division of obturator nerve, L2–L4.

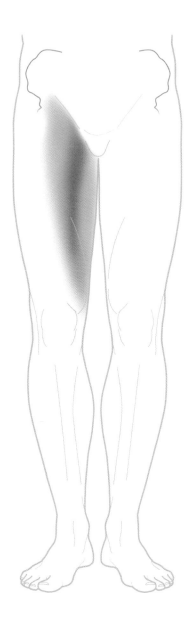

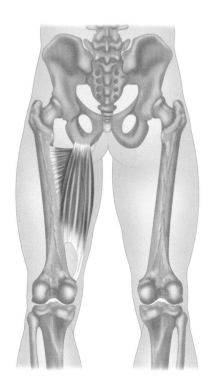

Muscle name
Adductor magnus.

Latin, *adductor*, toward; *magnus*, large.

Origin
Inferior or anterior ramus of pubis in angle between crest and symphysis (anterior fibres). Ischial tuberosity (posterior fibres).

Insertion
Entire length of femur extending from the gluteal tuberosity along the linea aspera, medial supracondylar line, and adductor tubercle on medial condyle of femur.

Kinetic chain comment
Decelerates femoral external rotation and abduction of the thigh.

Trigger point comment
Pain referred from adductor magnus can manifest itself in many ways including deep pelvic pain, pubic, bladder, rectal, or vaginal pain. This pain can often be mistaken for serious visceral or gynaecological pathology. When pathology is not clear, trigger points should be investigated as the root cause of this severe pain.

Nerve
Tibial portion of sciatic nerve, L4, 5, S1. Posterior division of obturator nerve, L2–L4.

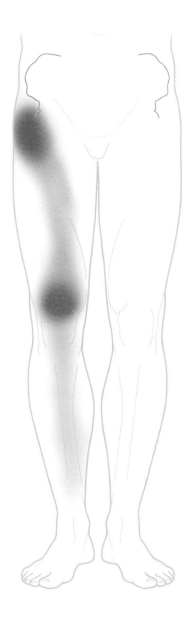

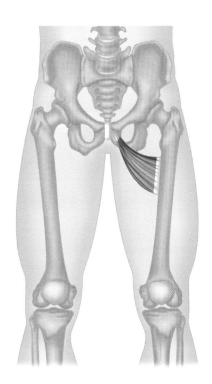

Muscle name
Adductor brevis.

Latin, *adductor*, toward; *brevis*, short.

Origin
Outer surface of inferior ramus of the pubis.

Insertion
On a line extending from lesser trochanter to upper part of linea aspera.

Kinetic chain comment
Decelerates femoral external rotation and abduction of the thigh.

Trigger point comment
Pain felt deep in the hip predominantly on the medial side of the thigh and referring to the medial aspect of the knee joint which can be mistaken for arthritic pain.

Nerve
Anterior division of obturator nerve, L2–L4.

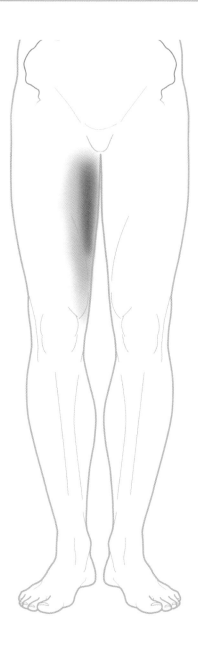

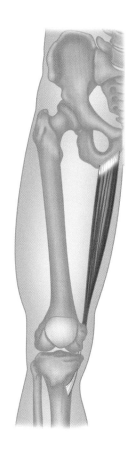

Muscle name
Gracilis.

Latin, *slender*, delicate.

Origin
Anterior lower half of symphysis pubis and medial margin of inferior ramus of pubis.

Insertion
Front and medial surface of the shaft of the tibia just below the condyle.

Kinetic chain comment
Decelerates femoral external rotation and abduction of the thigh.

Trigger point comment
Trigger points not only refer pain but also change in sensation. This muscle is a good example of that. Patients complain of a hot and stinging feeling on the inner thigh just superficial to the skin.

Nerve
Anterior division of obturator nerve, L2–L4.

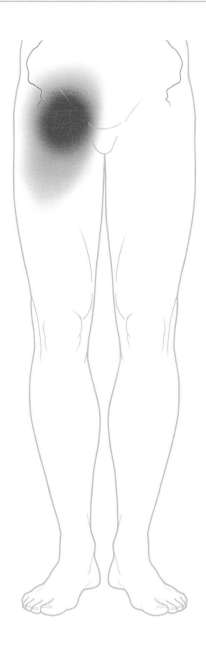

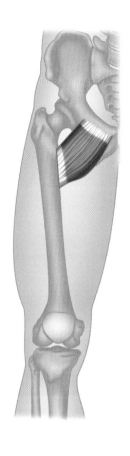

Muscle name
Pectineus.

Latin, *pecten*, comb; *pectenate*, shaped like a comb.

Origin
Pecten line of the pubis between the iliopubic eminence and pubic tubercle.

Insertion
Pectineal line of femur, from lesser trochanter to linea aspera.

Kinetic chain comment
Decelerates femoral external rotation and abduction of the thigh.

Trigger point comment
This pain is felt deeply in the groin as a sharp pain within the femoral triangle. Similar to the adductor muscle group, the pain is sometimes felt in the joint itself.

Nerve
Femoral and obturator nerves, L2–L4.

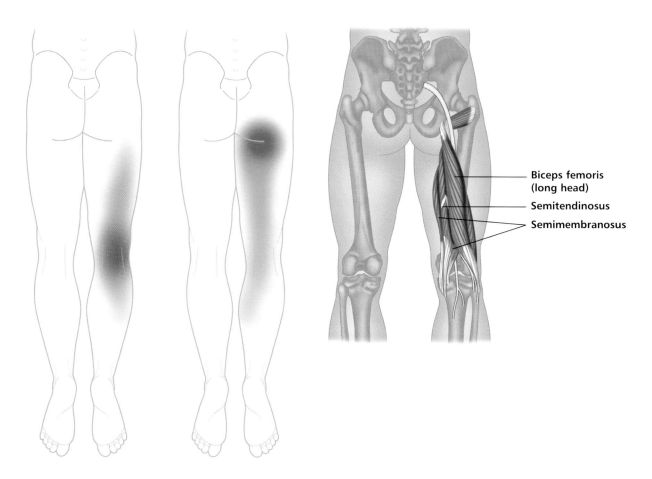

Biceps femoris
(long head)

Semitendinosus

Semimembranosus

Muscle group
Hamstrings (semimembranosus (SM), semitendinosus (ST), biceps femoris (BF)).

German, *hamme*, back of leg.

Origin
They all attach from the ischial tuberosity. Biceps femoris blends a long head with the sacrotuberous ligament and its short head attaches in the linea aspera and intermuscular septum.

Insertion
ST and SM attach to the posteromedial tibia by means of the tibial condyle (SM) and the medial surface of the tibia, including the deep fascia (ST).

Action
SM, ST and BF flex the knee joint. SM and ST medially rotate the knee joint and assist in medial rotation of the hip joint when the knee is flexed. BF laterally rotates the knee joint and assists in lateral rotation of the hip joint when the knee is flexed.

Kinetic chain comment
All the hamstrings eccentrically contract in gait to decelerate extension of the knee joint and hip flexion whilst playing a very important role in pelvic stability. They decelerate internal rotation on heel strike. The hamstrings disappear under the gluteus maximus and provide force closure of the sacroiliac joint with the coupled action of the force provided by the contra-lateral latissimus dorsi. This force is transmitted through the sacrotuberous ligament and further up to the thoraco-lumbar fascia. Short weak hamstrings can affect the erector spinae, multifidus, gluteus medius, or heel position and plantar fascia.

Trigger point comment
Typically pain is referred up towards the gluteals with some residual pain spreading down just below and behind the knee, even into the medial gastor of gastrocnemius. This pain can often be mistaken for sciatic pain. Weak inhibited gluteals, including medius, can lead to trigger points forming in the hamstrings and lumbar erector muscles including the quadratus lumborum. Ultimately the hamstrings are trying to become gluteals while the lumbar muscles are trying to be hamstrings. Is it any wonder hamstrings are such an injured muscle in sport?

Nerve
Sciatic nerve, L4, 5, S1–3.

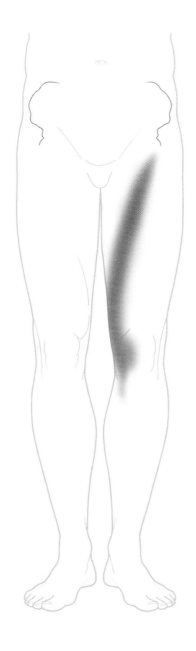

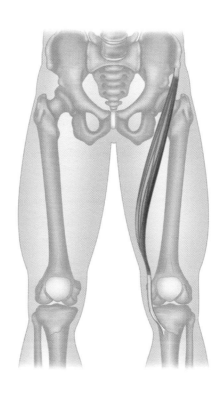

Muscle name
Sartorius.

Latin, *tailor*.

Origin
ASIS (anterior superior iliac spine).

Insertion
Superior aspect of the medial surface of the tibial shaft near the tibial tuberosity.

Action
Flexes and laterally rotates the hip joint and flexes the knee (tailor's muscle).

Kinetic chain comment
Sartorius decelerates extension and medial rotation at the hip joint and extension at the knee. Baby or satellite MtPs to consider include: rectus femoris, vastus medialis, pectineus, adductor longus, brevis and magnus.

Trigger point comment
A severe burning or sharp tingling pain or sensation is experienced along the anterior but mostly medial aspect of the thigh and knee cap. Typically this is not felt as a deep knee pain. Be sure to test for chondromalacia patellae (runner's knee).

A few words about vastus medialis obliquus

Some anatomists consider vastus medialis oblique fibres to be a separate and functionally distinct structure. These oblique fibres attach to the tendon of rectus femoris and medial border of the patella and the anterior medial condyle of the tibia. It is interesting to note the expansions that pass across the knee joint to attach to the tibia replace the joint capsule in this region, and then fuse with the deep fascia embracing the tibial tuberosity.

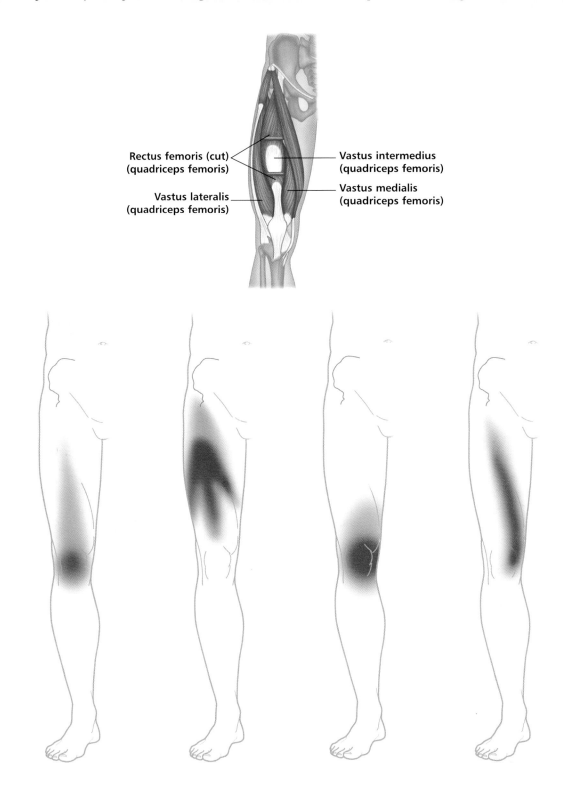

Rectus femoris (cut)
(quadriceps femoris)

Vastus intermedius
(quadriceps femoris)

Vastus lateralis
(quadriceps femoris)

Vastus medialis
(quadriceps femoris)

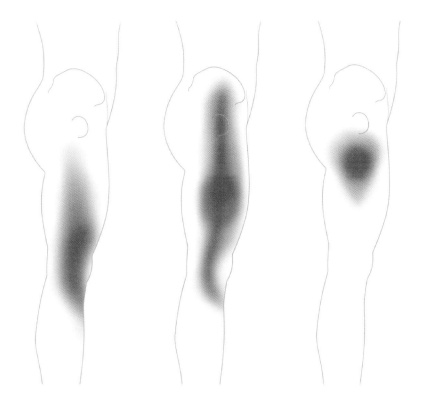

Muscle group
Quadriceps (rectus femoris, vastus medialis, vastus lateralis, vastus intermedius).

Latin, four-headed; **Greek**, four-footed.

Origin
Rectus femoris originates from the anterior inferior iliac spine (AIIS) and from the groove above the rim of the acetabulum.

Vastus medialis originates from the anterior intertrochanteric line, medial lip of the linea aspera, and proximal aspect of the medial supracondylar line. It is interesting to note the attachment into tendons of adductor longus and magnus and into the medial intermuscular septum.

Vastus lateralis originates from the intertrochanteric line and the greater trochanter, gluteal tuberosity and lateral lip of the linea aspera and the lateral intermuscular septum.

Vastus intermedius originates on the anterior lateral surface of the proximal two-thirds of the femur, the distal half of the linea aspera and the lateral intermuscular septum.

Articularis genu: Two slips from anterior femur below vastus intermedius (pulls capsule superior).

Insertion
All of the quadriceps muscles wrap-up the patella (sesamoid bone) with each having a unique and specific line of pull or directional force acting on the patella.

They share a common tendon (patellar tendon or ligament) and attach to the tibial tuberosity.

Action
Extends the knee joint. Rectus femoris additionally flexes the hip joint.

Kinetic chain comment
These muscles contribute a significant influence on pelvic rotation (anterior), on knee cap tracking and knee positioning. Shortness in the quadriceps can ultimately affect head and neck positioning, cause knee pain, and affect foot and ankle movement. Eccentric contraction decelerates knee flexion, adduction, and internal rotation on heel strike of the gait cycle. Rectus femoris eccentrically decelerates hip extension and knee flexion during gait. The inter-relationship of all the quadriceps provides dynamic stability to the knee.

Trigger point comment
A multitude of trigger points have been identified within the quadriceps group. It may seem strange, but typical pain involves a deep toothache-like pain (vastus medialis) in the knee joint, or on the lateral or medial aspect of the thigh including the knee. My tip based on clinical experience concerning knee pain is to check for trigger points in the muscles of the mouth if no success is achieved with treatment and/or exercise.

Nerve
Femoral nerve, L2–4.

Muscles of the Hip and Thigh

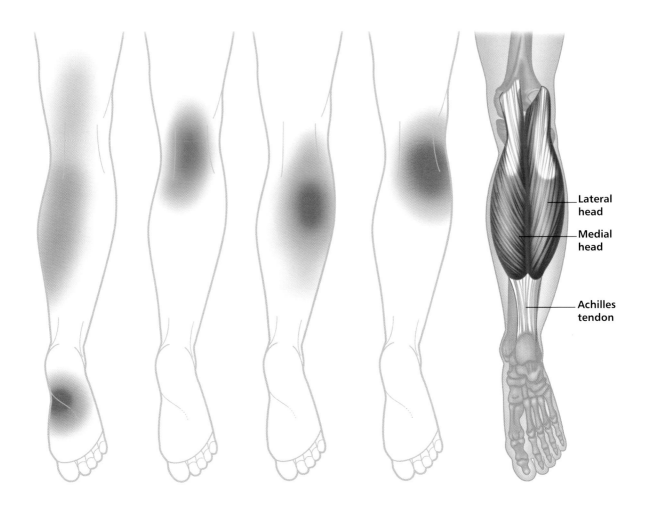

Lateral
head

Medial
head

Achilles
tendon

Muscle name
Gastrocnemius.

Greek, *gaster*, stomach; *kneme*, leg.

Origin
Medial and lateral condyles of the femur (posteriorly) and from the capsule of the knee joint and oblique popliteal ligament.

Insertion
Posterior surface of the calcaneus (heel bone).

Action
Running or walking, gastrocnemius provides considerable forces, enough to propel our bodies in jumping. A powerful plantar flexor, it contracts eccentrically to assist deceleration of femoral internal rotation and assists in external rotation of the knee during the push-off phase and aids knee flexion during the swing of gait.

Kinetic chain comment
The relationship with the heads of the gastrocnemius and tendons of the hamstrings must be considered when participating in machine-based exercise. A shared fascia with the plantar muscles of the foot can highlight the need for balance, both up and down the kinetic chain. Eccentrically it decelerates ankle extension in gait.

Trigger point comment
Several trigger points can form in this muscle referring pain and a sense of stiffness or tension into the medial plantar aspect of the foot and diffuse pain spread over one or both of the gastors. Pain can also refer up into the medial hamstrings. Typically individuals will try to statically stretch the symptoms away. This will irritate the muscle spindle response and serves only to compound the symptoms. The posterior kinetic chain should be assessed to identify short hypertonic muscles and myofascial migration.

Nerve
Tibial nerve, S1, 2.

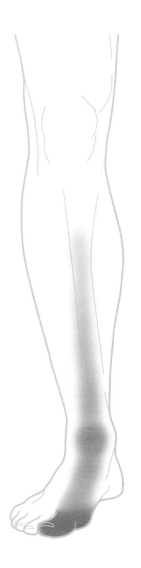

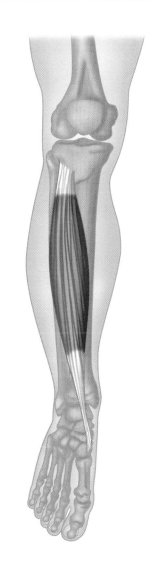

Muscle
Tibialis anterior.

Latin, *tibia*, pipe or flute / shinbone; *anterior*, before.

Origin
Lateral condyle and proximal two-thirds of lateral surface of the tibia, interosseous membrane, deep fascia and lateral intermuscular septum.

Insertion
Medial and plantar surface of medial cuneiform bone, base of metatarsal bone.

Action
Dorsiflexes the ankle joint and assists in inverting the foot. When contracting eccentrically, it decelerates plantar flexion at heel strike and eversion of the mid-foot in mid-stance. It offers dynamic stabilization to the mid-tarsal joint and accelerates supination of the foot before heel strike.

Kinetic chain comment
Due to the reciprocal inhibition, tibialis anterior can become weak, long and tight, predisposing the foot to over pronation and eversion (flat foot). Short, spastic or contractured peroneals will facilitate this inhibition reducing soft tissue support to all three foot arches.

Trigger point comment
Trigger points in tibialis anterior refer down into the big toe. Pain can also be experienced in the ankle (anteromedially) as it passes the retinaculum. Fallen arches in the foot place eccentic loads on tibialis anterior while hypercontracted peroneals will increase inhibition to tibialis anterior. All in all, a recipe for trigger point evolution.

Nerve
Deep peroneal nerve, L4, 5, S1.

A few words to identify other muscles involved with plantar flexion

Flexor hallucis longus and flexor digitorum longus are deep muscles of the posterior compartment of the lower limb attaching all the way down to the toes. Plantar flexion also involves the tibialis posterior. Together these muscles are called Tom, Dick and Harry. The plantaris is a muscle with a small gastor, yet it has the longest tendon in the human body. Situated on the lateral condyle of the femur it runs down to attach to the calcaneus sharing the common calcaneal tendon with gastrocnemius and soleus.

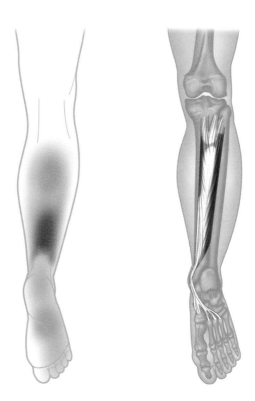

Muscle name

Tibialis posterior.

Latin, *tibia*, pipe or flute/shinbone; *posterior*, behind.

Origin

Upper half of the lateral aspect of the posterior surface of the tibia, most of the interosseous membrane, posterior fibula and the fascia covering it posteriorly.

Insertion

Tuberosity of navicular and plantar surface of the medial cuneiform. Tendinous expansions attach to the plantar surfaces of all the tarsal bones (except the talus) and the tip of the sustentaculum tali and the bases of the middle three metatarsals.

Action

Plantar flexion and inversion (supination). Eccentrically it decelerates subtalar joint pronation as it controls subtalar eversion, internal rotation of the tibia and dynamically stabilizes the talonavicular joint. In push-off phase of gait, it assists in plantar flexion and inversion.

Kinetic chain comment

This muscle dives deep into the sole of the foot, the foundation upon which we all stand. Due to reciprocal inhibition, tibialis posterior can neurologically weaken leading to compromised arch support. This can have implications further up the chain to links such as popliteus, posterior intermuscular septum, adductor magnus, and the core musculature.

Trigger point comment

Most people will mistake the trigger points in tibialis posterior for Achilles tendonitis, plantar fasciitis, or shin splints. Pain is felt on the medial tibia or in the sole of the foot, at the level of the arch, on walking. Clients will often present with a pronated foot. A functional kinetic chain assessment is required with appropriate activity to improve core stability and kinetic chain integrity.

Nerve

Branch of the tibial nerve, L4, 5, S1.

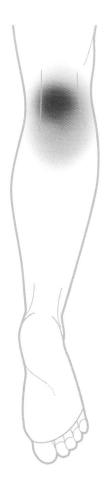
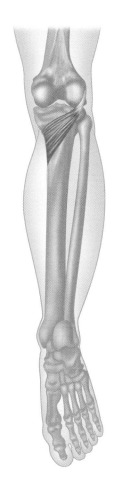

Muscle name
Popliteus.

Latin, *poples*, ham.

Origin
Anterior aspect of the lateral condyle of the femur and oblique popliteal ligament of the knee joint. It is anchored by a strong tendon to the lateral condyle of the femur to the capsule of the knee joint and can include the lateral meniscus.

Insertion
Posterior surface of the posterior side of the proximal tibia above the soleal line.

Action
Medially rotates the tibia on the femur and flexes the knee (non-weight bearing). When the feet are fixed (closed chain kinetics) it laterally rotates the femur on the tibia and flexes the knee joint. Eccentrically it decelerates tibial rotation internally and femoral rotation externally (screw home effect). Its function in posterolateral stability is significant. Some anatomical papers describe a common idea of the popliteus as a retractor of the lateral meniscus.

Kinetic chain comment
Machine-based exercise such as prone leg curls can overstress popliteus causing spasm and diminished screw home capability. This in turn can lead to an inhibited piriformis and deep hip rotators with hyperextension at the knee. Shortness can be confirmed by observing slight flexion and internal rotation of the anatomical leg.

Trigger point comment
This muscle is one that takes a lot of stressful abuse and eventually trigger points form causing pain in the back of the knee. At night the pain reduces or ceases completely. Stiffness in the knee joint is often evident in the morning with reduced ability to fully extend the anatomical leg. On assessment, the foot can look like the leg has turned in (medial rotation at the knee). This is often as a result of heavy squat exercises in the absence of appropriate neuromuscular stability at the joints and within the core.

Nerve
Tibial nerve, L4, 5, S1.

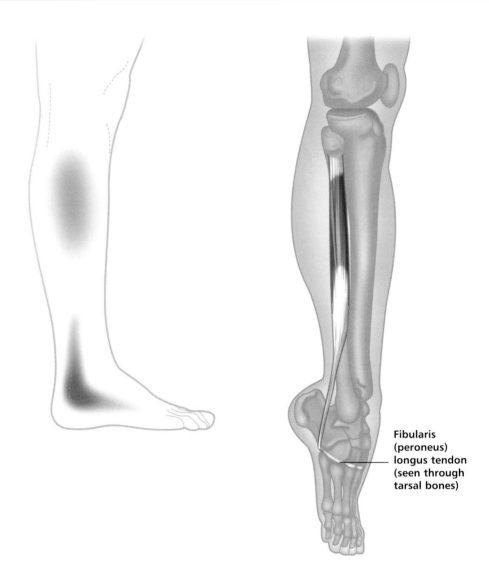

Fibularis (peroneus) longus tendon (seen through tarsal bones)

Muscle name
Fibularis (peroneus) longus.

Latin, *fibula*, pin/buckle; *longus*, long.

Origin
Lateral condyle of the tibia (in conjunction with extensor digitorum longus) upper two-thirds of the lateral surface of the fibula, intermuscular septa and the deep fascia.

Insertion
Plantar and lateral surface of the medial cuneiform and base of the first metatarsal.

Action
A foot evertor, it assists with plantar flexion of the ankle joint. It depresses the head of the first metatarsal. It eccentrically decelerates ankle dorsiflexion and inversion of the subtalar joint during the push-off phase of gait.

Kinetic chain comment
This muscle forms a sling or stirrup for the foot arches offering opposing force to tibialis anterior. Further up the kinetic chain it can affect the function of the biceps femoris, sacrotuberous ligament, erector spinae, multifidus, etc.

Trigger point comment
Along with the peroneus brevis, trigger points refer pain down the leg over, above, and behind the lateral malleolus. Pain can also be felt over the anterolateral aspect of the ankle and outside of the calcaneus. Many individuals with these trigger points complain of numbness or pins and needles in the toes, especially the third and fourth toe and the big toe.

Nerve
Superficial peroneal nerve, L4, 5, S1.

A few words on plantaris

A long slender muscle owning the longest (Achilles) tendon in the body, its origin is on the lateral supracondylar ridge, popliteal surface and joint capsule. It inserts into the medial surface of calcaneus. It is a weak flexor of the knee and plantar flexes the ankle in the push-off phase of gait.

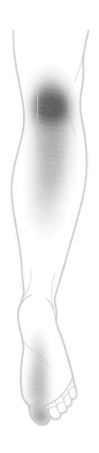
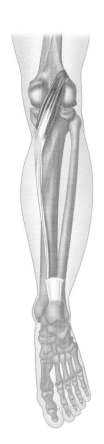

Muscle name

Plantaris.

Latin, *planta*, sole of the foot.

Origin

Inferior aspect of lateral supracondylar line of distal femur and oblique ligament of the knee.

Insertion

Middle third of the posterior surface of the calcaneus, medial to Achilles tendon.

Action

Plantar flexes the foot at the ankle, inversion and assists in flexion at the knee.

Kinetic chain comment

A weak contributor to decelerating extension of the knee joint and decelerating eversion and dorsiflexion at the ankle.

Trigger point comment

The pain from MtPs in plantaris mimics many pain syndromes firing into the posterior knee and down the medial aspect of the triceps surae into the heel and sometimes into the ball of the foot and the big toe. The therapist must rule out the possibility of S1 or S2 radiculopathy, rupture of the plantaris, popliteus tendinitis, tenosynovitis, popliteal artery aneurysm, Baker's cyst, deep vein thrombosis (DVT), intermittent claudication, peripheral vascular disease (PVD), avulsion of popliteus tendon, muscle strain, posterior compartment syndrome, popliteal lymphedema, systemic infections or inflammation, nutritional inadequacy, metabolic imbalance, toxicity, and possible side effects of medications.

Nerve

Tibial nerve, L4, 5, S1.

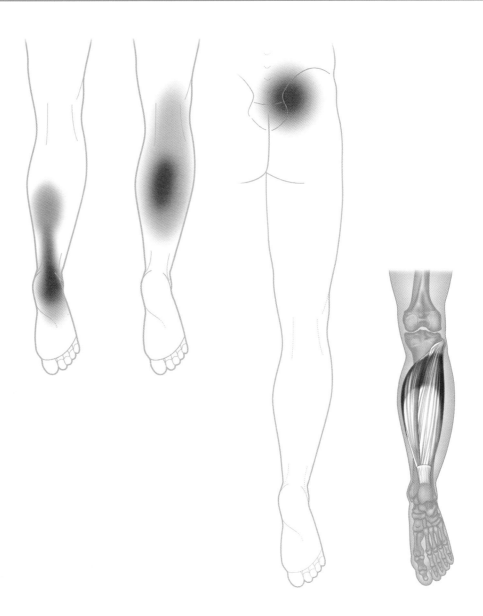

Muscle name
Soleus.

Latin, sole-shaped (fish).

Origin
(Lying deep to gastrocnemius). This broad flat muscle resembles a flat fish. From the soleal line on the medial border of the tibia, posterior surface of the upper third of the fibula and the fibrous arch between.

Insertion
By means of the calcaneal tendon to the middle part of the posterior surface of the calcaneus (heel bone).

Action
Along with the gastrocnemius and plantaris, it plantar flexes the ankle.

Kinetic chain comment
From a dynamic postural viewpoint, it prevents the body falling forwards at the ankle joint during standing. In gait, it eccentrically decelerates subtalar joint pronation and internal rotation of the lower leg at heel strike. Decelerates dorsiflexion of the foot. Spasm or trigger points in soleus can be the origin of tight hamstrings, low back pain, and even headaches.

Trigger point comment
Soleus typically refers pain into the posterior aspect and plantar surface of the heel and the distal end of the Achilles tendon. A rare trigger point spreads pain to the ipsilateral sacroiliac joint and also in extreme cases, pain can be referred to the jaw.

Nerve
Tibial nerve, L5, S1, 2.

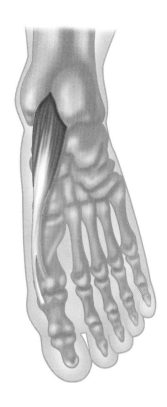

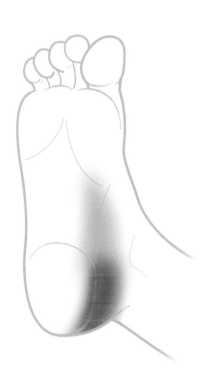

Muscle name
Abductor hallucis.

Latin, *abduct*, away from; *hallux*, great toe.

Origin
Along the medial tuberosity of the calcaneal bone, flexor retinaculum and the plantar aponeurosis.

Insertion
By means of the outer edge of the medial sesamoid, onto the medial base of the proximal phalanx of the big toe (hallux).

Action
Abduction and flexion of the metatarsophalangeal joint. Assists in adducting the forefoot.

Kinetic chain comment
Working with flexor hallucis brevis and longus and the adductor hallucis longus (to control the big toe), abductor hallucis belongs to the first layer of muscles on the foot. It decelerates adduction of hallux at the metatarsophalangeal joint (eccentric control towards the anatomic axis of the foot). Failure to do this leads to increasing pronation of the big toe and progression of the deformity.

Trigger point comment
Pain is felt in the medial and posterior portions of the heel as well as the instep. This can be experienced as a burning sensation on heel strike and toe off. Patients tend to limp into the clinic. Experience leads me to look at the footwear of my patients which are often too small or fit badly. Be sure to rule out contributions from the possibility of L4 radiculopathy, S2 sciatic nerve lesion, Achilles tendinitis, plantar fasciitis, bone spur, pes cavus, pes planus (flat feet), bunions, congenital hypertrophy, Morton's foot syndrome, diabetic neuropathy, polyneuropathy, reflex sympathetic dystrophy, bone fracture, sprain/strain, tarsal tunnel syndrome, callus, involvements of blisters, bursitis, osteoarthritis, and rheumatoid arthritis. If in doubt, refer.

Nerve
Medial plantar nerve, L4, 5, S1.

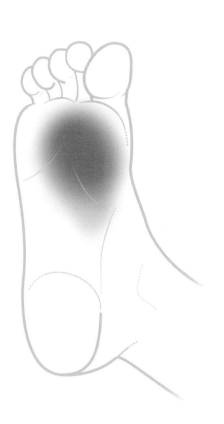

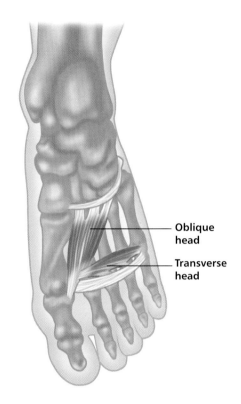

Oblique
head

Transverse
head

Muscle name
Adductor hallucis.

Latin, *adduct*, toward; *hallux*, great toe.

Origin
Two heads (oblique and transverse) attach this muscle from bases of the second to the fourth metatarsal bones, plantar metatarsophalangeal ligaments of the third through to the fifth digits and deep transverse metatarsal ligament.

Insertion
Lateral side of base of proximal phalanx.

Action
Adducts and assists in flexing the metarsophalangeal joint of the big toe.

Kinetic chain comment
Implicated as a major deforming factor in hallux valgus, the adductor hallucis decelerates movement of the proximal phalanx away from the second toe and also decelerates the lateral sesamoid reducing further pronation. Failure to do so adequately is a potent cause of the more severe hallux valgus deformity.

Trigger point comment
The referral pattern is local with pain felt on the distal sole under the metatarsal heads. Patients often report numbness. A frequently used patient description is a feeling of 'fullness' in the area.

Nerve
Lateral plantar nerve, S1, 2.

Chaitow, L., and DeLany, J.: 2002. *Clinical Applications of Neuromuscular Techniques*. Churchill Livingstone, Edinburgh

Chaitow, L.: 2006. *Muscle Energy Techniques, Positional Release and Modern Neuromuscular Techniques*. Churchill Livingstone, Edinburgh

Chaitow, L. 1976. *The Acupressure Treatment of Pain*. Thorsons, London

Clemente, C. M. (editor): 1985. *Gray's Anatomy of the Human Body, 38th edition*. Lea & Febiger, Philadelphia

Course notes and syllabus content, National Qualification in Neuromuscular Therapy (Certificate and Higher Diploma level), National Qualification in Exercise and Health Studies (NCEHS) and National Qualification in Medical Pilates, Higher Diploma Medical Exercise Specialist, National Training Centre, Dublin, Ireland

Hsieh, Y L, et al.: 2007. Dry Needling to a Key Myofascial Trigger Point May Reduce the Irritability of Satellite Myofascial Trigger Points. *Am. J. Phys. Med. Rehabil.*, **86**, 397–403

Ingber, D. E.: 2006. Mechanical Control of Tissue Morphogenesis During Embryological Development. *Int. J. Dev. Biol.*, **50**, 255–266, American Academy of Osteopathy

Jarmey, C.: 2003. *The Concise Book of Muscles*. Lotus Publishing/ North Atlantic Books, Chichester/ Berkeley

Jones, L. H.: 1981. *Strain and Counterstrain*. Newark, Ohio

Niel-Asher, N.: 2005. *The Concise Book of Trigger Points*. Lotus Publishing/ North Atlantic Books, Chichester/ Berkeley

Sharkey, J.: 2003. The Stretching Debate. *J. of Bodywork and Movement Therapies*, 7, **2** (commentary 9), 90–93

Shier, I.: 2004. Does Stretching Improve Performance? A Systematic and Critical Review of the Literature. *Clinical Journal of Sport Med.*, **14**(5): 267–273

Travel, J. and Simons, D. 1999. *Myofascial Pain & Dysfunction: the Trigger Point Manual (vol. 1, 2nd edn.)*. Lippincott, Williams & Wilkins, Baltimore

Travel, J. and Simons, D. 1993. *Myofascial Pain & Dysfunction: the Trigger Point Manual (vol. 2)*. Lippincott, Williams & Wilkins, Baltimore

Various. *Journal of Bodywork and Movement Therapy (JBMT)*. Churchill Livingstone, Edinburgh

General Index

Abduction	20, 52, 87
Acceleration	60
Acetabulum	20
Acetylcholine (ACh)	81
Actin	70, 73, 81
Action of muscles	66
Active trigger points	80, 83
Acute	20
Adduction	20, 52, 87
Adenosine diphosphate (ADP)	76
Adenosine monophosphate	76
Adenosine triphosphate (ATP)	25, 26, 74, 76, 81
Adhesions	20
Afferent	20
Afferent cells, *see sensory cells*	
Agonists	53, 66, 100
Amphiarthrotic joints	32
Analogous	20
Anatomical localization	20
Anatomical position	20
Anatomy, understanding	17
Anomaly	20
Antagonists	53, 66, 100
Anterior	20
Anterior sagittal chain	104
Anterior tilt	20
Aponeurosis	20, 64, 71
Appendicular skeleton	23, 28
Arndt-Schultz's law	115
Arthrokinematics	59, 62, 85, 88
Articulation	20
Associative stage	97
Atrophy	107
Attachment trigger points	83
Autonomous stage	97
Avascular necrosis	37
Axial skeleton	23, 28
Axon	41
Baby trigger points, *see satellite trigger points*	
Balance	91
Bind	124
Biomechanics, *see arthrokinematics*	
Bipennate muscles	66
Blood	44
Blood pressure	46
Border	35
Bursa	64
Cardiac cycle	44, 45

Cardiac muscle	62
Cardiac output	46
Cardiorespiratory	44
Cardiovascular system	43
Cartilage	28
Caudal	20
Cell	25
Cellular metabolism	26
Central trigger points	82, 83
Chronic	20
Circumduction	52
Citric acid cycle, *see Kreb's cycle*	
Client records	111
Co-contraction	100
Cognitive stage	96
Combining forms	18
Compression	60
Condyle	35
Connective tissue	38, 39
Connective tissue lock	130
Connective tissue release	130
Contracture	80
Contraindications	84, 119
Contralateral	20
Contrary points methodology	126
Coracoid	35
Core stability	96
Coronal plane, *see frontal plane*	
Cranial	20
Creams	131
Crest	35
Critical fibre distance	38, 71
Cross-bridge cycling	74
Crosstalk	122
Davis' law	116
Deep	20
Deep anterior chain	104
Dendrite	41
Depression	52
Dermatome	20
Diathrotic joints	32
Diet	37, 83
Directional force	100
Displacement	60
Distal	21
Dorsal	21
Dorsiflexion	52
Dynamic balance	92
Dynamic neutral	127, 128

Dysfunction 49
Dyskinesis 89

Ease 124
Eccentric contraction 53, 74
Efferent 21
Efferent cells, *see motor cells*
Effleurage 114
Electron transport chain 27
Elevation 52
Embryogenesis 48
Endomysium 71
Endosteum 35
Energy 60, 76
Epicondyle 35
Epimysium 71
Epiphyses 35
Epitendineum 64
Equine neuromuscular therapy 51
Eukaryotic cells 25
Evagination 21
Eversion 52
Excretion 25
Extension 21, 52, 87
Extracellular matrix (ECM) 38, 48

Facilitation 122
Fascia 21, 48, 105
Fascicles 71
Fast twitch fibres 129
Fat 50
Fine motor skills 77
Flexion 21, 52, 87
Fluid 60
Foramen 21, 35
Force 60
Force closure 106
Force couple relationships 59
Form closure 106
Fossa 21, 35
Free nerve endings 91
Friction 21
Frontal plane 21, 51, 53, 112
Fulcrum 67
Functional trigger points 86

Galea aponeurosis 49
Ganglion 21
General adaptation syndrome 107
Glenohumeral internal
    rotation deficit (GIRD) 89
Glycogenolysis 27
Glycolysis 27
Golgi tendon organs 41, 91

Gradual increments of contraction 76
Greater trochanter 21
Gross motor skills 77
Growth 25

Head's law 116
Hilton's law 116
Histiocyles 38
Homeostasis 27, 46
Hooke's law 116
Horizontal plane, *see transverse plane*
Hydrosis 128
Hydrostatic pressure 60
Hypertrophy 107

Individual difference 111
Induration technique 128
Inferior 21
Inflammation 107
Inhibition 55
Insertion 21, 64
Integrated neuromuscular
    inhibition technique (INIT) 122, 128
Intermediate 21
Interneuron 54
Inversion 52
Ipsilateral 21
Irritability 25
Ischemic pressure 128
Isolytic contraction, *see isotonic eccentric*
Isometric contraction 53, 118, 128
Isotonic concentric 118
Isotonic eccentric 118

Joint 21

Key trigger points 83
Kinesthetic awareness 93
Kinetic chain 53, 100, 101
Knee jerk stretch, *see patellar tendon stretch*
Kreb's cycle 27

Lactates 27
Lacunae 28
Latent trigger points 80, 83
Lateral 21, 51
Lateral chain 102
Lateral rotation 87
Lateral scapular slide test 89
Law of facilitation 106, 115
Law of generalization 115
Law of intensity 115
Law of radiation 115
Law of symmetry 115

Law of unilaterality   115
Levers   67, 68
Ligament   21
Line of pull, *see directional force*
Local adaptation syndrome   107
Lotions   131
Lumbo-pelvic-hip complex   101, 111
Lumen   21

Macrophages   38
Mass   60
Massage   114
Mastoid   35
Meatus   21
Mechanoreceptors   92, 93
Mechnotherapy   131
Medial   21, 51
Medial rotation   87
Median   21
Median plane, *see mid-sagittal plane*
Medical exercise   95
Medullary cavity   35
Mid-sagittal plane   51, 112
Mitochondrion   25
Momentum   60
Monosynaptic reflex arc   41, 55
Motor   21
Motor cells   41
Motor units   76
Movement   25
Multipennate muscles   66
Muscle cell   72
Muscle control   97
Muscle energy techniques   118
Muscle fibre arrangement   62
Muscle function   105
Muscle shapes   65, 66
Muscle spindles   41, 54, 91
Muscle units   96
Muscular tone   76
Myelin sheath   42
Myocardium   45
Myofibrils   72
Myofilaments   72
Myokinetic chains   102
Myosin   70, 73, 81
Myosin cross-bridges   73

Nervous system   40
Nervous tissue   41
Neurolemma   42
Neuromuscular efficiency   62
Neuromuscular technique   117
Neurons   41

Neutralizers   53
Nodes of ranvier   42
Nodule   81
Notch   35
Nucleus   25

Oblique plane   51
Oils   131
Olecranon   49
Organelles   25
Origin   64
Osteonecrosis, *see avascular necrosis*
Oxidation   27
Oxidative decarboxylation   27

Palmar   21
Palpate   21
Parietal pleura   49
Patellar tendon stretch   55
Patent   21
Pathophysiology   95
Patient assessment   108
Perception   96
Perimysium   71
Periosteal vessels   36
Periosteum   35, 71, 105
Petrissage   114
Phasic component   55
Piezoelectric activity   38
Planes of motion   51
Plantar   21, 52
Plasma membrane   25
Plexus   21
Positional release   120, 123
Posterior   21
Posterior sagittal chain   103
Postganglionic   21
Post-isometric relaxation   118
Postural assessment-kinematic
    chain evaluation   112
Postural considerations   112
Precise motor skills, *see fine motor skills*
Prefixes   18
Preganglionic   21
Prevertebral   21
Primary afferent muscle spindle response   121
Primary trigger points   83
Prime movers   100
Process   21, 35
Progressive overload   110
Pronation   52
Prone   21
Proprioception   92, 93

Proprioceptive neuromuscular facilitation
　　stretching (PNF)　58
Protection　44
Protrusion　52
Proximal　21
Pulsed MET　119
Pyruvate　27
Ramus　35
Raphe　64
Reactive postural responses (RPR)　92
Reciprocal inhibition　61, 118, 124
Reflex arc　55
Regional areas　23
Regulation　44
Reproduction　25
Respiration　25
Retrusion　52
Reversibility　110
Ribose　76
Rotation　21, 52
Ruffini cells　91

Sagittal plane　22, 51, 53
Sarcolemma　71, 72
Sarcomere　56, 72, 80
Sarcoplasmic reticulum　72, 73
Satellite trigger points　80, 82, 83
Scapular assistance test　89
Scapular platform　88
Scapular retraction test　89
Sensory　22
Sensory cells　41
Septum　22
Serum hormone binding globens (SHBGs)　37
Sesamoid bones　30, 64
Sharkey's spray and stretch　129
Shear　60
Sherrington's law　61, 116
Shoulder anatomy　85
Shunt　66
Skeletal muscle　62
Skeletal system　28
Skin　50
Sliding filament theory　70, 73
Slow twitch fibres　129
Smooth muscle　62
Soft tissue release, see connective tissue release
Specificity　110
Spillover　121
Spin　66
Spine　35
Spiral chain　102
Spiralized muscles　66
Sprays　131

Stabilization　101
Stabilizers　53, 100
Stacking　127
Stages of learning　96
Static balance　92
Static dynamic　55
Static stretching　56
Strain　60
Strain/counterstrain　120
Strap muscles　66
Stress　60
Stretch reflex arc　58
Stroke volume　46
Styloid　35
Suffixes　18
Sulcus　91
Superficial　22
Superior　22
Supination　52
Supine　22
Swing　66
Synapse　81
Synarthrotic joints　32
Synergistic dominance　62
Synergists　53
Synovial joints　33

Tapotement　114
Target zone　82
Tendon　22, 64, 71
Tensile　60
Tension　60
Thoraco-lumbar gain　53
Titin　70, 73
Tonic component　55
Transportation　44
Transverse plane　22, 51, 53, 112
Transverse tubules　72
Trendelenberg's sign　88
Trigger point formation theories　81
Triplanar　106
Trochanter　35
Tropomyosin　73
Troponin　73, 74
True visceral pain　84
T tubules, see transverse tubules
Tubercle　22, 35
Tuberosity　22, 35

Unidirectional　106
Upper crossed syndrome　119

Valgus position　22
Variation　110

Varus position	22
Vasoconstriction	46
Vasodilation	46
Velocity	60
Ventilation	46
Ventral	22
Volar	52
Volkmann's canals	36
Weight	60
Wolff's law	116
Working environment	82

Index of Muscles

Abductor digiti minimi	192	Flexor digitorum superficialis	187
Abductor hallucis	227	Flexor pollicis longus	187
Abductor pollicis brevis	191	Frontalis	134
Abductor pollicis longus	189		
Adductor brevis	213	Gastrocnemius	220
Adductor hallucis	228	Gemellus inferior	207
Adductor longus	211	Gemellus superior	207
Adductor magnus	212	Geniohyoideus	140
Adductor pollicis	188	Gluteus maximus	202
Anconeus	185	Gluteus medius	203
		Gluteus minimus	204
Biceps brachii	181	Gracilis	214
Biceps femoris	216		
Brachialis	183	Iliacus	164
Brachioradialis	193	Infraspinatus	171
		Intercostales externi	157
Coracobrachialis	182	Intercostales interni	157
Deltoideus	180	Latissimus dorsi	179
Diaphragm	158	Levator scapulae	176
Digastricus	142	Longissimus capitis	154
		Longus capitis	144
Epicranius (occipitofrontalis), *see occipitalis/frontalis*		Longus colli	143
Erector spinae	151	Masseter	135
Extensor carpi radialis brevis	194	Multifidis	155
Extensor carpi radialis longus	195	Mylohyoideus	140
Extensor carpi ulnaris	196		
Extensor digitorum	197	Obliquus capitis inferior	149
		Obliquus capitis superior	150
Fibularis (peroneus) longus	224	Obliquus externus abdominis	160
Flexor carpi ulnaris	198	Obliquus internus abdominis	159
Flexor digitorum profundus	187	Obturator externus	209

Obturator internus   208
Occipitalis   134
Omohyoideus   141
Opponens pollicis   200

Palmaris longus   201
Pectineus   215
Pectoralis major   177
Pectoralis minor   169
Piriformis   206
Plantaris   225
Platysma   139
Popliteus   223
Pronator quadratus   190
Pronator teres   186
Psoas major   163
Psoas minor   165
Pterygoideus lateralis   138
Pterygoideus medialis   137
Pyramidalis, *see rectus abdominis*

Quadratus femoris   210
Quadratus lumborum   166

Rectus abdominis   162
Rectus capitis anterior   145
Rectus capitis lateralis   145
Rectus capitis posterior major   148
Rectus capitis posterior minor   148
Rectus femoris   219
Rhomboideus major   168
Rhomboideus minor   168
Rotatores   156

Sartorius   217
Scalenus anterior   146
Scalenus medius   146
Scalenus posterior   146
Semimembranosus   216
Semitendinosus   216
Serratus anterior   175
Soleus   226
Splenius capitis   152
Splenius cervicis   153
Sternocleidomastoideus   147
Sternohyoideus   140
Sternothyroideus   140
Stylohyoideus   140
Subclavius   178
Subscapularis   173
Supinator   199
Supraspinatus   170

Temporalis   136
Tensor fasciae latae   205
Teres major   174
Teres minor   172
Thyrohyoideus   140
Tibialis anterior   221
Tibialis posterior   222
Transversus abdominis   161
Trapezius   167
Triceps brachii   184

Vastus intermedius   219
Vastus lateralis   219
Vastus medialis   219

The Anatomy of Stretching

Brad Walker

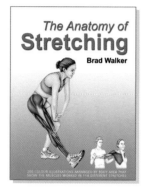

978 1 905367 03 0 (UK)/978 1 55643 596 (US); **£14.99/$24.95**; 176 pages; 265 mm x 194 mm; 320 colour illustrations; paperback

Books on stretching are common, but *The Anatomy of Stretching* takes a more fundamental approach than the others, taking the reader inside the body to show exactly what is happening during a stretch. At the heart of the book are 300 full-colour illustrations that show the primary and secondary muscles worked in 114 key stretches arranged by body area. Author Brad Walker brings years of expertise – he works with elite-level and world-champion athletes, and lectures on injury prevention – to this how-to guide. He looks at stretching from every angle, including physiology and flexibility; the benefits of stretching; the different types of stretching; rules for safe stretching; and how to stretch properly. Aimed at fitness enthusiasts of any level, as well as at fitness pros, *The Anatomy of Stretching* also focuses on which stretches are useful for the alleviation or rehabilitation of specific sports injuries.

Brad Walker, B.Sc. Health Sciences, is a prominent Australian sports trainer with more than 20 years experience in the health and fitness industry. He graduated from the University of New England, and has postgraduate accreditations in athletics, swimming, and triathlon coaching.

The Anatomy of Sports Injuries

Brad Walker

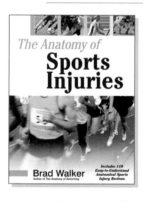

978 1 905367 06 1 (UK)/ 978 1 55643 666 6 (US); **£16.99/$29.95**; 256 pages; 265 mm x 194 mm; 250 colour / black and white illustrations; paperback

The Anatomy of Sports Injuries takes you inside the body to show exactly what is happening when a sports injury occurs. At the heart of *The Anatomy of Sports Injuries* are 300 full-colour illustrations that show the sports injury in detail, along with 200 line drawings of simple stretching, strengthening, and rehabilitation exercises that the reader can use to speed up the recovery process. *The Anatomy of Sports Injuries* is for every sports player or fitness enthusiast who has been injured and would like to know what the injury involves, how to rehabilitate the area, and how to prevent complications or injury in the future. This book is the perfect partner for Brad's other book, *The Anatomy of Stretching*.

Brad Walker, B.Sc. Health Sciences, is a prominent Australian sports trainer with more than 20 years experience in the health and fitness industry. He graduated from the University of New England, and has postgraduate accreditations in athletics, swimming, and triathlon coaching.

Dynamic Bodyuse for Effective, Strain-free Massage

Darien Pritchard

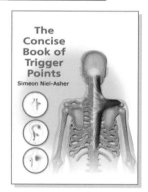

978 0 9543188 9 5 (UK)/ 978 1 55643 655 0 (US); **£24.99/$39.95**; 640 pages; 265 mm x 194 mm; 2000 black and white photographs; paperback

The most significant cause of early retirement from the massage profession is the *cumulative strain* on the body developed in the course of performing massages. The growth of the profession in recent years has been accompanied by an increase in the number of work-induced problems. This book highlights aspects of massage that can lead to these problems and offers guidance for their avoidance. The focus is on how to use your body *safely* and *effectively* in massage sessions. This includes *involving your whole body* to generate the power and movement that supports your working hands, *saving your hands* by using them skilfully, and *conserving them* by using other body areas such as your forearms and elbows whenever possible. This book is essential reading for anyone involved in massage, whether you are a student, a professional massage practitioner or teacher, or sports massage therapist.

Darien Pritchard calls upon over 30 years of training massage professionals. He also teaches bodywork modules in a university degree course, and has written a series of articles for *Massage World* on bodyuse.

The Concise Book of Trigger Points

Simeon Niel-Asher

978 0 9543188 5 7 (UK)/ 978 1 55 643 536 2 (US); **£16.99/$29.95**; 208 pages; 275 mm x 212 mm; 260 colour / black and white illustrations; paperback

Written for the student and early practitioner of massage / bodywork, physical therapy, physiotherapy, and any other health-related field. It explains how to treat chronic pain through trigger points. Each two-page spread has colour illustrations of each major skeletal muscle, and text identifying each muscle's origin, insertion, action, and innervation, plus the physiological implications of the trigger points in each muscle, and techniques for treatment.

Simeon Niel-Asher, B. Phil., B.Sc., (Ost.), qualified as an osteopath in 1992. He is involved in treating, research, writing, and teaching throughout Europe, the Middle East, and the USA.

"This book represents an excellent entry level text which will be a powerful learning aid to any student or newly qualified practitioner."
John Sharkey, B.Sc., Neuromuscular Therapist, Director, National Training Centre, Ireland